Publishing Your Medical Research Paper

What They Don't Teach in Medical School

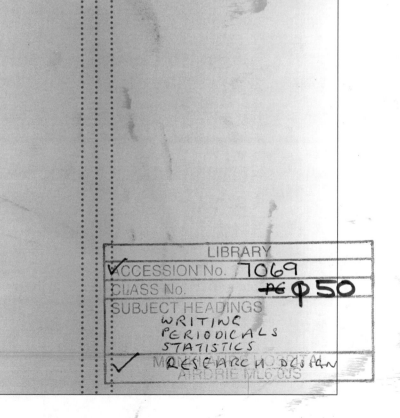

...eturn on or before the last ...hown belo...

Publishing Your
Medical Research Paper

*What They Don't Teach
in Medical School*

....

Daniel W. Byrne

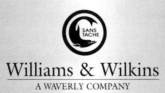

Williams & Wilkins
A WAVERLY COMPANY

BALTIMORE • PHILADELPHIA • LONDON • PARIS • BANGKOK
BUENOS AIRES • HONG KONG • MUNICH • SYDNEY • TOKYO • WROCLAW

Editor: Elizabeth Nieginski
Manager, Development Editing: Julie Scardiglia
Managing Editor: Darrin Kiessling
Marketing Manager: Rebecca Himmelheber
Development Editor: Rosanne Hallowell
Production Coordinator: Felecia Weber
Designer: D. Pfisterer
Illustration Planner: Felecia Weber
Cover Designer: D. Pfisterer
Typesetter: Peirce Graphic Services, Inc.
Printer/Binder: Transcontinental Printing, Inc.

Copyright © 1998 Williams & Wilkins

351 West Camden Street
Baltimore, Maryland 21201–2436 USA

Rose Tree Corporate Center
1400 North Providence Road
Building II, Suite 5025
Media, Pennsylvania 19063–2043 USA

All terms mentioned in this book that are known to be trademarks or service marks have been appropriately capitalized. Williams & Wilkins cannot attest to the accuracy of this information. Use of a term in this book should not be regarded as affecting the validity of any trademark or service mark. The publisher cannot guarantee the suitability or accuracy of information, or the availability of resources listed in this book. All information contained herein is subject to change. Mention of a specific product or company does not imply an endorsement.

This book is not part of Mark H. McCormack's series: *What They Don't Teach You at Harvard Business School* and *What They Still Don't Teach You at Harvard Business School.*

Background research for this book was not sponsored by or affiliated with The Journal of the American Medical Association or any other journal mentioned in this book.

Please use the following information when citing this book:
Byrne DW. *Publishing Your Medical Research Paper: What They Don't Teach in Medical School.* Baltimore, MD: ©1998 Williams & Wilkins.

Printed in Canada

Library of Congress Cataloging-in-Publication Data

Byrne, Daniel W.
  Publishing your medical research paper : what they don't teach in medical school / Daniel W. Byrne. — 1st ed.
     p.   cm.
  Includes bibliographical references and index.
  ISBN 0–683–30074–1
  1. Medical writing.   2. Medicine—Research—Methodology.
  I. Title.
  R119.B97   1997
  808'.06661—dc21   97-29896
                                                                              CIP

The publishers have made every effort to trace the copyright holders for borrowed material. If they have inadvertently overlooked any, they will be pleased to make the necessary arrangements at the first opportunity.

To purchase additional copies of this book, call our customer service department at **(800) 638–0672** or fax orders to **(800) 447–8438.** For other book services, including chapter reprints and large quantity sales, ask for the Special Sales department.

Canadian customers should call **(800) 665–1148,** or fax **(800) 665–0103.** For all other calls originating outside of the United States, please call **(410) 528–4223** or fax us at **(410) 528–8550.**

Visit Williams & Wilkins on the Internet: http://www.wwilkins.com **or contact our customer service department at** custserv@wwilkins.com**. Williams & Wilkins customer service representatives are available from 8:30 am to 6:00 pm, EST, Monday through Friday, for telephone access.**

                                                                98 99 00
                                                1 2 3 4 5 6 7 8 9 10

To Loretta, Michael, and Virginia

Contents

List of Tables

List of Figures

Preface

"Worship the spirit of criticism," Pasteur advised his fellow scientists. Today, most scientists recognize the importance of this advice, but nearly all prefer the spirit of praise from one particular group: peer reviewers. The bad news is that each year reviewers reject hundreds of thousands of medical manuscripts. The good news is that many are rejected for common flaws that can be avoided.

Several books have described how to write a scientific paper, notably those by Robert Day (1994), Edward Huth (1990), and George Hall (1994). My goal in writing *Publishing Your Medical Research Paper: What They Don't Teach in Medical School* was to explain how to anticipate and avoid the problems typically encountered in designing a research study and writing a publishable paper.

Many common reviewer criticisms can be avoided simply by understanding the research and publishing processes and by following certain fundamental principles. This book presents 245 principles in five sequential phases: **P**lanning, **O**bserving, **W**riting, **E**diting, and **R**evising. Applying these **POWER** principles will increase the likelihood that your research will be accepted for publication. The information in this book will also help you critically assess new medical information and extract what you need to know.

As background research for this book, I surveyed a number of experts, including editors-in-chief of prominent medical journals, peer reviewers from the *Journal of the American Medical Association,* and recent Nobel Prize winners. Additionally, I analyzed hundreds of actual reviews to identify common themes and distilled specific comments into positive guidance. These ideas are arranged into 245 principles presented in an easy-to-read format, with short examples of actual peer review critiques. To protect the privacy of those involved, some of these comments are paraphrased or generalized.

Publishing Your Medical Research Paper is designed for those who want to publish their work without spending endless amounts of money on epidemiologists, computer consultants, statisticians, technical writers, and graphic artists. It provides an organized collection of solutions to help you publish your medical research paper. For those who manage a team of research specialists, these solutions will help you stretch your research dollar. Although this book focuses on clinical research, most of the principles can also be applied to nonclinical subjects.

This book does not attempt to explain everything you need to know about statistical analysis, epidemiology, or writing. For more complex problems, I have recommended an appropriate specialist or a specific book. To help you obtain this information, I have included a directory of telephone numbers and Internet Web site addresses in Appendix D. Special icons used throughout the book are as follows:

 Actual peer reviewer comments about a manuscript

 Comment from survey respondents

◎ VITAL POINT: Advice emphasized by many experts

⊕ FOR MORE INFORMATION: Experts, books and Internet Web sites

Academic publishing requires time, dedication, practice, and, above all, persistence. If you can muster these resources, you will be rewarded with seeing your article in print and knowing that your work has made a difference. As Anne Roe said: "Nothing in science has any value to society if it is not communicated."

— Daniel W. Byrne

Acknowledgments

All published work and quotations are referenced as accurately as possible. As promised, the survey responses were kept anonymous, but I am nonetheless grateful to the reviewers and editors who completed and returned my questionnaires. Also, the many anonymous journal peer reviewers who work so hard are impossible to thank by name, but I do appreciate the time and effort they volunteered.

Dr. Gertrude Elion and Mr. Robert Jacoby were kind enough to read and find something nice to say about early drafts of this book. To Mr. Paul van Niewerburgh I express deep gratitude for his support and encouragement. For more than a decade he has generously shared his writing expertise with me. Despite a hectic schedule he found time to critique and edit many drafts of this manuscript. His wisdom and hard work have significantly improved both the writing and content of this book. I am indebted to Dr. Jane Petro for her encouragement and excellent research material. Thanks to Dr. Harold Horowitz for his perceptive critiques, to Dr. Jean Morgan for the expert advice, Dr. Albert Lowenfels for his encouragement and important ideas, to Ms. Chris Hunter for sharing her knowledge of the Internet, to Dr. Lawrence Wexler, Dr. Luis Bracero, Dr. P.D. Reddy, Mr. Evan Jones, and Dr. Michael Blumenfield. My family deserves special thanks, especially Bill Byrne, Karen Peach, Jim Byrne, Ed and Jane May, and Tom and Loretta Byrne.

I gratefully acknowledge the professional assistance of the people at Williams & Wilkins, especially Ms. Elizabeth Nieginski, Ms. Julie Scardiglia, Ms. Karla Schroeder, Ms. Rosanne Hallowell, Ms. Beth Goldner, and Ms. Jacqueline Jenks. Also, I'd like to extend my thanks to the numerous reviewers contacted by Williams & Wilkins for their valuable editorial comments and suggestions.

Finally, but most of all, a special thanks to my wife, Loretta, for her thoughtful suggestions and endless patience.

CHAPTER 1.

Overview: Ten Key Principles

Your success in publishing your medical research paper will largely depend on how well you follow these ten key principles. Study these points before moving on to the more detailed principles and periodically review these key principles during your research project.

PRINCIPLE 1. INVEST AMPLE TIME AND MONEY IN PLANNING.

"Just do it!" may be a successful slogan for selling sneakers, but it's a poor approach to conducting medical research. You need both an experienced research team and an extensive literature review to avoid the common problems encountered in planning the study protocol, designing the measures of outcome, creating the data collection form, and performing the statistical analysis.

PRINCIPLE 2. FORMULATE YOUR STUDY PROTOCOL EARLY.

The study protocol is the written plan for your research project. A good protocol provides direction, focus, and structure. As you conduct your study, follow this plan and document all decisions and developments. This approach allows you to monitor and describe the accuracy and appropriateness of your methods. Keep the protocol and all papers related to the study organized into binders.

PRINCIPLE 3. DESCRIBE YOUR METHODS THOROUGHLY.

To show that your findings can be applied to larger populations, clearly describe your sample and study design. Readers and reviewers will scrutinize your methods before they accept your conclusions.

PRINCIPLE 4. DESCRIBE THE RATIONALE FOR THE SIZE AND COMPOSITION OF YOUR SAMPLE.

Explain how and why you chose to study this number of patients. Discuss the implications and statistical power of your decision. Help the reader to understand your logic in selecting this group of patients for the study.

PRINCIPLE 5. EXPLAIN WHAT IS NEW, INTERESTING, AND USEFUL ABOUT YOUR RESULTS.

What do your findings contribute to the medical literature? Explain the importance of the research problem and your findings for both physicians and patients.

PRINCIPLE 6. KEEP THE MANUSCRIPT SHORT.

Plan to submit a paper that is 10% shorter than the average article in your target journal. Check the total length of the paper, the length of each section, and the number of references. Use fewer tables and figures than average.

PRINCIPLE 7. ANSWER THE QUESTIONS: "SO WHAT?" AND "WHO CARES?"

Emphasize the points that distinguish your study from other research. Your paper must contain sections anticipating negative reactions from reviewers. Remember that to be accepted, your subject must interest most of your target journal's readers.

PRINCIPLE 8. FOLLOW THE GUIDELINES AND FORMAT OF THE TARGET JOURNAL PRECISELY.

Consult the information for authors and several recent issues of the target journal. Be sure that your submission meets the journal's definition of a complete manuscript. Also consider the timeliness of the subject from the perspective of the target journal's readers.

PRINCIPLE 9. EDIT RUTHLESSLY.

Ask colleagues in your laboratory or department to read your paper objectively. Continue to revise your manuscript until it is both clear and polished. Write an introduction that captures the reader's attention, and rewrite the remaining text as necessary to maintain the reader's interest.

PRINCIPLE 10. WRITE CAUTIOUS, BUT PERCEPTIVE CONCLUSIONS.

Devote the necessary time and effort to writing quality conclusions. Your conclusions must be insightful and clearly justified. They should include a smooth, logical transition from your results, and end with a bang!

P L A N N I N G

P
O
W
E
R

Key Questions to Answer in the Planning Phase:

- *What is the research problem?*

- *What is the plan to study this problem?*

- *How can this study benefit patient care?*

CHAPTER 2.

Methods: Laying the Groundwork

CHOOSING A TOPIC

PRINCIPLE 11. CHOOSE A TOPIC THAT IS TIMELY, IMPORTANT, AND INTERESTING.

The ten key principles discussed in Chapter 1 outline the process of writing an article for publication, but the remaining 235 principles provide the all-important details. Obviously, the first step in planning is to select a research topic.

How do you select a topic for study? Your interest in and passion for a research topic should be the prime motivators. However, since you also are planning to publish your results, you must understand how the journal publishing process works and consider where your topic fits in.

First, you must consider the target audience. You can begin by asking yourself two questions:

1. Is my main research question important and interesting to enough readers?
2. Do I have the resources to answer this question?

A research project demands a significant investment of time, so you must be genuinely interested in the topic and internally motivated to complete the project. However, the key to getting your study published is the **importance of the topic**. A common reason for rejection is simply a lack of importance. For this reason, choose a topic that has clinical interest, but keep your study **simple**. When you find an interesting problem, consider studying and presenting a solution. In this way, the focus of your study will be on the solution, not the problem.

If you are a novice at writing papers, seek advice from an experienced investigator, mentor, or department chairperson who can help you select a worthwhile research project with a publishable slant.

◎ VITAL POINT

Early in your project, solicit opinions of other researchers and an experienced statistician. They can help you avoid many pitfalls.

A classic mistake of the inexperienced researcher is waiting until the study is nearly completed to ask for help.

⊕ FOR MORE INFORMATION

See *Designing Clinical Research* by Hulley and Cummings (1988) and also *Healthy People 2000* (US Public Health Service, 1991), which provides a detailed account of the United States government's health goals for the year 2000 (see Appendix D).

CONDUCTING A LITERATURE SEARCH

When you review the literature, do not be intimidated by the work that has been published. Much of the medical literature is flawed or outdated, so be skeptical. By studying the literature carefully, you often can design a study that is superior to those already published. Although your work should not duplicate published reports, do not hesitate to continue your research if someone has published a paper that initially looks like a barrier to your progress, because many publications are not as strong as they initially appear.

You can use an online service, such as Grateful Med, Ovid Technologies, PaperChase, Physicians' Online, or The UnCover Company, to conduct a literature search from your home or office personal computer (see Appendix D).

You also can have a full-text copy of an article mailed or faxed directly to you through a document delivery service (see the Institute for Scientific Information, Knight-Ridder, Ovid Technologies, SilverPlatter, and The UnCover Company in Appendix D). When using any of these services, you will see the following two acronyms:

- MEDLARS: the MEDical Literature Analysis and Retrieval System, maintained by the United States National Library of Medicine (NLM).
- MEDLINE (MEDlars onLINE): one of more than 40 online databases within MEDLARS. MEDLINE contains approximately 8 million articles and abstracts from 4000 biomedical journals published since 1966.

Another option is a CD-ROM literature searching system, such as the systems available from Aries Systems, EBSCO, Knight-Ridder, Ovid Technologies, or SilverPlatter (see Appendix D). CD-ROM literature searching systems, such as SilverPlatter, are available at many medical libraries and may be the best place to begin. A reference librarian can show you how to select search terms. As you may already have discovered, learning how to conduct a literature search on the Internet takes practice, but is worthwhile.

⊕ FOR MORE INFORMATION

See Appendix D for telephone numbers and Internet Web sites. Some services provide free MEDLINE access, but ask the reference librarian at your medical library for the latest information on these services. If you have no idea where to start, try PubMed. See the US National Library of Medicine in Appendix D.

REDUNDANT AND MULTIPLE PUBLICATIONS

One important principle to keep in mind in the early planning stage is never to submit a paper that is a redundant publication or a duplicate publication. As one expert warned: **"Avoid cutting a single study into a large number of small parts"**. In other words, do not stretch one natural paper into several trivial papers with overlapping results. Another expert said: "Multiple manuscripts that could have been submitted as one manuscript were not received well by the editor or the reviewers, and if the papers were not rejected outright, the authors were requested to combine the manuscripts into one concise manuscript." One reviewer advised: "Make a contribution to mankind, not just to your curriculum vitae."

⊕ FOR MORE INFORMATION

See the following sections in Appendix A: "Redundant or Duplicate Publication" and "Acceptable Secondary Publication."

PRINCIPLE 12. UNDERSTAND WHAT REVIEWERS CONSIDER A "GOOD" ARTICLE.

You can increase the likelihood that your paper will be accepted by learning what reviewers look for in submissions.

Table 2–1 shows the responses of reviewers who were asked to define a good article.

Table 2–1. Reviewers' Responses to the Question: "What Is Your Definition of a Good Article?"*
— One that makes the reader wonder: "Why didn't I think of that?"
— Deals with an important, interesting, and contemporary topic: the aim is clearly stated; the methodology is correct; the study is well presented and has a concise, interesting discussion
— Relevant to the audience and clinical practice
— Original
— Results should be reproducible
— Good design of experiments to answer a specific question that has not already been answered in the literature
— Adequate discussion of the shortcomings of the design and conclusion
— Tight, clear organization
— Clear, easy-to-read communication that teaches or stimulates ideas in the reader
— Omits irrelevant points
* From question 30 of the Peer Review Questionnaire in Appendix B.

FORMING A RESEARCH TEAM

PRINCIPLE 13. JOIN OR FORM A RESEARCH TEAM WITH THE RIGHT CHEMISTRY.

For an established researcher, the first step in performing a study is to recruit a research team. To produce high-caliber science, experienced investigators have learned that a team must have the right blend of skills and personalities. They choose people who have a reputation for doing their share of the work and avoiding academic politics.

When you participate in assembling a research team, select people who will work well together and show respect for one another (e.g., by coming to meetings on time). Check references, and talk with candidates' previous research teams. Seek team members who have the free time and motivation to complete the project; a famous scientist or department chairperson may not be the most suitable person for the job. Although a well-known investigator's reputation and connections may help your paper to get noticed, remember that many journals use a "blinded" system in which authors' names are not used during the review process.

The most productive medical research teams often are composed of highly skilled and experienced people with a variety of academic degrees (master's, bachelor's, and nursing as well as doctoral and medical).

Choosing the right person to collect the data can be a challenge. Data collection often is more time-consuming than anticipated, and the ideal person for this task must have sufficient time. For this reason, hiring a full-time research nurse may be more efficient than persuading a harried medical student or resident to collect data. Also remember that many research projects require more than one person to collect data.

The ideal data collection person for a clinical research project has the following characteristics:

- Pays attention to detail
- Follows instructions precisely
- Asks questions when unsure
- Is not overcommitted with other responsibilities
- Remains objective
- Has years of experience in the medical field

Recruit at least one team member who is a talented writer. **Discuss authorship early and candidly.** Do not assume that any member of a research team will, or will not, be a coauthor of your study. Authorship depends on a "substantial contribution to the intellectual content of the study," so never list an author who has not met the full criteria for authorship.

⊕ FOR MORE INFORMATION

See Appendix A for a full description of the authorship standards established by the International Committee of Medical Journal Editors.

Consider asking the person who collects the data and the statistician to coauthor the paper. Coauthorship motivates many people to do their best work. In addition, many studies hinge on the quality of the work of these two people, and some public accountability is logical. Moreover, readers have the right to know who collected and analyzed the data.

You do not have to be a chairperson with a $5 million grant to form a research team. Medical students, residents, and junior faculty who have no budget or authority can form a research team by diplomatically asking the right people to collaborate. If you are polite and hardworking, many experts will work with you on worthwhile projects. Remember that today you can form a "virtual research team" of experts from around the world by using modern technology. However, be sure that this team also has the right chemistry.

CHAPTER 3.

The Methodology

PRINCIPLE 14. STATE THE PROBLEM.

The top priorities in the planning stage are:

- **Conceptualizing the problem**
- **Formulating a good approach to solving the problem**

Conceptualizing a clinical research problem requires you to organize your thoughts and draw general conclusions from specific instances. Only when the problem and aim of the study are thought out and concisely defined can you begin to collect data. **Ask your colleagues to critique your methodology, and make the recommended changes, which you agree with, before you begin to collect data.**

Adherence to traditional scientific methodology is essential. The steps in the scientific method are as follows:

1. State the problem.
2. Formulate the hypothesis.
3. Design the study.
4. Collect data.
5. Interpret the data.
6. Draw conclusions.

STATING THE PROBLEM

Stating the problem is the first and most important step in the scientific method. The idea for a problem may come from anecdotal observations, the literature, ongoing or previous research, conferences, or conversations with colleagues. Whatever the source of the idea, quality research requires a polished problem statement. You must be able to provide a clear and concise answer to the question: "What is the main purpose of this study?"

Example 3–1.

Approximately 40% of patients with spinal cord injury develop a pressure ulcer during the initial hospitalization. However, there is currently no method of quantifying this risk that is accurate for this population.

FORMULATING THE HYPOTHESIS

PRINCIPLE 15. FORMULATE YOUR HYPOTHESIS.

After you state the problem, the next step in the scientific method is to formulate the hypothesis. The *American Heritage Dictionary* (1996) provides a nice definition of a hypothesis: "a tentative explanation that accounts for a set of facts and can be tested by further investigation."

Many experienced researchers prefer to start with the null hypothesis (H_0), which is a clear, testable statement about chance occurrence that assumes no difference or association between two variables. Typically, the assumption involves an association between risk factors and outcome or a difference in outcome between patients who receive one treatment versus another. For example:

1. A history of cigarette smoking is not associated with the incidence of lung cancer.
2. Preoperative serum albumin level is not associated with the occurrence of postoperative complications.
3. The infection rate will not be significantly different between patients given drug A and patients given drug B.

The alternative hypothesis (H_A) is the opposite of the null hypothesis. Your research team should jointly develop at least one null hypothesis and several alternative hypotheses before you begin to collect data. Scrutinize these hypotheses and the major goals of the study, and lay down the criteria to reject the null hypothesis. Discuss as many alternative hypotheses as possible with the research team.

⊕ FOR MORE INFORMATION

Chapter 12 of Hulley and Cummings (1988).

DESIGNING THE STUDY

PRINCIPLE 16. **RESEARCH THE STRONGEST APPROPRIATE STUDY DESIGN.**

The third step in the scientific method is to design the study. Obviously, different medical research problems require different types of studies. For the typical clinical study of treatment, however, first attempt to use what commonly is considered the ideal design (Table 3–1).

This ideal design is not always possible; for example, clinical evaluation of the course of a disease cannot be "triple-blinded." Still, to achieve your objectives, use the strongest appropriate study design.

The study design needs a good methodology. Do not underestimate the importance of planning. You can strengthen your study during the planning phase by addressing problems that cannot be corrected after the data are collected.

◎ VITAL POINT

A common flaw at this stage of a research project is lack of originality in study design.

Table 3–1.   Ideal Clinical Research Study Design

✔A sample that is:

- Large enough to answer the research question
- Homogeneous for the topic or research question
- Representative of a broad population
- Drawn from several different hospitals (multicenter)

✔An intervention that is:

- Randomized
- Placebo-controlled (patients in the control group receive an inactive substance)
- Evaluated in a dose-response method (see principle 63)
- "Triple-blinded" (patients, clinicians, and statisticians are unaware of which group is subject to which intervention)

✔A measure of outcome that is:

- Well defined
- Specific
- Objective
- Widely accepted as a measure of success
- Directly observed by an independent observer
- Based on long-term, quality-of-life variables (ideally from questionnaires answered by patients)
- Measured prospectively (see principle 17)
- Recorded as part of a comprehensive database, along with all potentially confounding factors, and quantified or coded properly

STUDY DESIGN TERMINOLOGY

PRINCIPLE 17. MASTER STUDY DESIGN TERMINOLOGY.

Figure 3–1 shows that study design flaws are the most important type of general flaw to avoid. Figures 3–2 and 3–3 provide more specific information to help you anticipate the most common and serious problems. The first step in improving your odds of publication is understanding the different types of study designs. The following terms are often misunderstood:

- Incidence
- Prevalence
- Exposure

Incidence is the number of **new** cases of a disease in a defined population over a specific period.

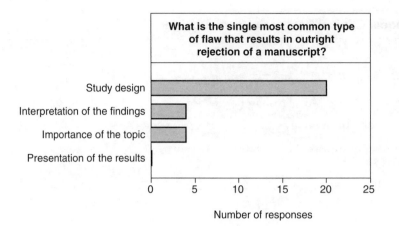

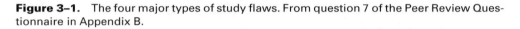

Figure 3–1. The four major types of study flaws. From question 7 of the Peer Review Questionnaire in Appendix B.

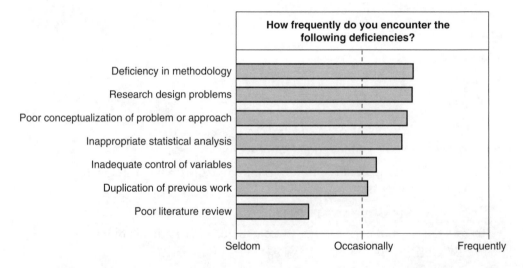

Figure 3–2. The frequency of certain study deficiencies. Answers are ranked by the mean using the following values: 0 = never; 1 = seldom; 2 = occasionally; 3 = frequently; 4 = always. From question 19 of the Peer Review Questionnaire in Appendix B.

Example 3–2.

In 1996, the number of new cases of HIV infection in residents of New York City was X per 100,000.

Prevalence is the total number of cases of a disease **existing** in a given population at a specific time.

Example 3–3.

The number of cases of HIV infection on January 1, 1997, was Y per 100,000 residents of New York City.

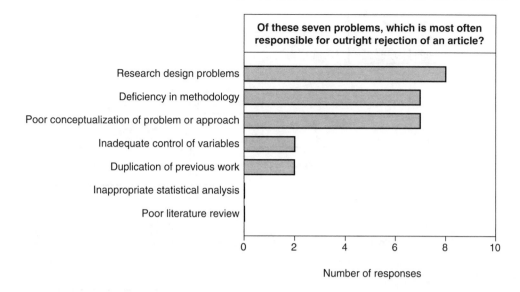

Figure 3–3. Study deficiencies that often are responsible for rejection. From question 20 of the Peer Review Questionnaire in Appendix B.

Prevalence depends on the incidence and duration of the disease. For highly lethal diseases, mortality rate also must be considered. These variables are interrelated as follows:

$$Prevalence = (Incidence - Mortality\ rate) \times Duration$$

⊕ FOR MORE INFORMATION

See Rothman (1986).

Exposure describes whether a person was physically subjected to a suspected cause (an etiologic factor). For instance, among passengers of a cruise ship, *exposure* might be defined as those who used the ship's hot tub. In clinical research, *exposure* often describes the presence of a characteristic or preexisting condition, such as diabetes.

Study designs can be classified most simply as follows:

1. Descriptive studies
2. Analytic studies

Study designs can also be classified more specifically into the following categories:

1. Observational studies
2. Quasi-experimental studies
3. Experimental studies

Figure 3–4 shows a flowchart of study designs.

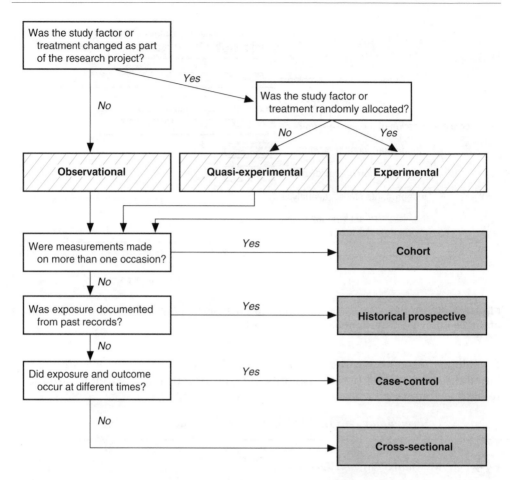

Figure 3–4. Flowchart of study designs. These questions refer to what the investigators did as part of this research project.

Descriptive studies report the frequency of conditions and the characteristics of the study population.

Analytic studies examine the relation between variables to detect risk factors and make inferences.

Observational studies are those in which the experience or exposure to a factor is observed, not manipulated.

Example 3–4.

Researchers compare newborn infants from two groups. In one group, the mothers used cocaine during pregnancy. In the other group, the mothers did not use cocaine during pregnancy.

In *quasi-experimental studies,* a study factor or treatment is changed, but the change is not randomly allocated.

Example 3–5.

Researchers compare the outcome of infants born in two cities. In one city, a new law was enacted to test pregnant women for cocaine use and enroll those who had positive test results in a treatment program. The other city had no such law or program.

Experimental studies actively change the exposure with an intervention, then measure the effect on an outcome. Experimental studies are stronger for proving causation.

Example 3–6.

Researchers compare newborn rats from two groups. In one group, the researchers had given the mothers cocaine during pregnancy. The mothers of the rats in the other group were not given cocaine during pregnancy.

PRINCIPLE 18. CHOOSE THE OPTIMAL DESIGN FOR YOUR STUDY.

The four major types of research studies (Figure 3–5) are as follows:

1. Case-control studies
2. Cohort studies
3. Historical prospective studies
4. Cross-sectional studies

Case-control studies (also known as case-referent or retrospective studies) use two groups of subjects: those with and those without a disease. The history of these two groups is studied to determine whether differences between them could help to explain why the disease developed in one group. The investigators then try to determine whether previous exposure or a particular attribute is responsible for the development of the disease.

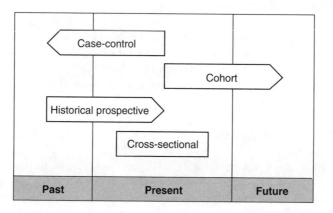

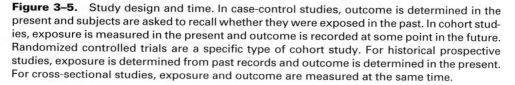

Figure 3–5. Study design and time. In case-control studies, outcome is determined in the present and subjects are asked to recall whether they were exposed in the past. In cohort studies, exposure is measured in the present and outcome is recorded at some point in the future. Randomized controlled trials are a specific type of cohort study. For historical prospective studies, exposure is determined from past records and outcome is determined in the present. For cross-sectional studies, exposure and outcome are measured at the same time.

In case-control studies, the study participants with the disease are obviously the cases, but choosing a control group is a challenging task. By definition, control subjects are members of the reference group: they do not have the disease, but are drawn from a population similar to the group with the disease.

Example 3–7.

Food poisoning develops in one-third of the guests at a wedding reception. Investigators question all of the guests about what they ate at the reception. The results are compared between the cases (with the food poisoning) and the controls (those without food poisoning).

In clinical research, most case-control studies are more complex, such as in the following example:

Example 3–8.

Orthopedic surgeons find that pneumonia develops in 6.6% of patients admitted to the hospital with a hip fracture. The surgeons want to test the hypothesis that the pneumonia is related to a history of exposure to passive smoking. On discharge from the hospital, they interview all patients who had a hip fracture about the duration and amount of exposure to passive smoking. They then compare the patients who had pneumonia with those who did not to determine whether there is a difference that would be unlikely to result from chance. They probably would also try to match the patients who did not have pneumonia with those who did on the most obvious variables, such as age, sex, type of fracture, and procedure, to be sure these factors are not responsible for the observed differences.

Case-control studies can be completed in less time and for less money, and ordinarily are more efficient than studies that follow patients over time. Case-control studies are useful for studying rare conditions and conditions with long intervals between exposure and outcome.

These studies often are called "retrospective" studies, but the term "retrospective" is ambiguous and should be avoided as a label for the design of a study. However, writing that a researcher "retrospectively reviewed medical records after the patients were discharged from the hospital" is acceptable.

⊕ FOR MORE INFORMATION

See Chapter 7 of Hulley and Cummings (1988) and the books by Sackett et al. (1991) and Spilker (1991).

Cohort studies also are known as follow-up, prospective, or incidence studies. They take measurements over time in a group of people, and they track new cases of a disease. Study subjects are classified by exposure status and are followed to determine whether the disease develops. Cohort studies are time-consuming, expensive, and often inadequate for rare conditions. They are effective for proving causation, measuring incidence, assessing the course of a condition, and studying conditions that cause sudden death.

Longitudinal studies (occasionally called "diachronic studies") are a type of cohort study in which subjects are followed over time to observe the natural course of a disease. These studies do not always use a control group. Although the term "prospective" is sometimes used to describe this type of study, this term can be confusing and should be avoided for labeling the overall study design. "Prospective cohort study" is clear, but "prospective study" is too vague.

Randomized controlled trials (also called "intervention studies," "experimental studies," or "randomized clinical trials"; Table 3–2) are another form of cohort study and ordinarily are considered the strongest study design. They are considered the strongest because the prevalence of potential confounding factors, even those that the researchers are unaware of, should be similar in the placebo group and the treatment group. Because of the randomization procedure, these two groups should, for example, have similar numbers of smokers. Therefore, randomization can often simplify the statistical analysis.

Randomized controlled trials are excellent for proving causation. Over the years, many ethical randomized controlled trials have been conducted that have contributed greatly to our understanding of medicine. Often, however, the ideal randomized study is not ethical for research in humans.

⊕ FOR MORE INFORMATION

See the *JAMA* Instructions for Authors (*JAMA* 1997; 277:74–82).

Historical prospective studies identify a group of people, then determine from past records whether they were exposed to a certain factor or had a particular attribute. Researchers determine whether, after that baseline point, the outcome of interest occurred. "Retrospective cohort studies" are better described as "historical prospective studies."

Example 3–9.

A registry was created of trauma patients who were admitted to a hospital. After each patient was discharged or died, a research nurse reviewed the hospital chart. Baseline factors, recorded on admission to the hospital, were analyzed to determine whether they were predictive of complications that developed during the hospital stay. This investigation is a historical prospective study.

Table 3–2.   Checklist to Be Used by Authors When Preparing or by Readers When Analyzing a Report of a Randomized Controlled Trial

Item	Yes	No	Unable to Determine
✔ State the unit of assignment.	☐	☐	☐
✔ State the method used to generate the intervention assignment schedule.	☐	☐	☐
✔ Describe the method used to conceal the intervention assignment schedule from participants and clinicians until recruitment was complete and irrevocable.	☐	☐	☐
✔ Describe the methods used to separate the generator and executor of the assignment.	☐	☐	☐
✔ Describe an auditable process of executing the assignment method.	☐	☐	☐
✔ Identify and compare the distributions of important prognostic characteristics and demographics at baseline.	☐	☐	☐
✔ State the method of masking.	☐	☐	☐
✔ State how frequently care providers were aware of the intervention allocation, by intervention group.	☐	☐	☐
✔ State how frequently participants were aware of the intervention allocation, by intervention group.	☐	☐	☐
✔ State whether (and how) outcome assessors were aware of the intervention allocation, by intervention group.	☐	☐	☐
✔ State whether the investigator was unaware of trends in the study at the time of participant assignment.	☐	☐	☐
✔ State whether masking was achieved for the trial.	☐	☐	☐
✔ State whether the data analyst was aware of intervention allocation.*	☐	☐	☐
✔ State whether individual participant data were entered into the trial database without awareness of intervention allocation.	☐	☐	☐
✔ State whether the data analyst was masked to intervention allocation.	☐	☐	☐
✔ Describe fully the numbers and flow of participants, by intervention group, throughout the trial.	☐	☐	☐
✔ State the average duration of the trial, by intervention group, and the start and closure dates for the trial.†	☐	☐	☐
✔ Report the reason for dropout, by intervention group.	☐	☐	☐
✔ Describe the timing of measurements, by intervention group.	☐	☐	☐
✔ State the predefined primary outcomes and analyses.	☐	☐	☐
✔ Describe whether the primary analysis used the intention-to-treat principle.	☐	☐	☐
✔ State the intended sample size and its justification.	☐	☐	☐
✔ State and explain why the trial is being reported now.	☐	☐	☐

continued

Table 3–2.   Checklist to Be Used by Authors When Preparing or by Readers When Analyzing a Report of a Randomized Controlled Trial (*continued*)

Item	Yes	No	Unable to Determine
✔ Describe or compare trial dropouts and completers.	☐	☐	☐
✔ State or reference the reliability, validity, and standardization of the primary outcome.‡	☐	☐	☐
✔ Define what constituted adverse events and how they were monitored, by intervention group.	☐	☐	☐
✔ State the appropriate analytical techniques applied to the primary outcome measures.	☐	☐	☐
✔ Present appropriate measures of variability (e.g., confidence intervals for primary outcome measures).	☐	☐	☐
✔ Present sufficient simple (unadjusted) summary data on primary outcome measures and important side effects so that the reader can reproduce the results.	☐	☐	☐
✔ State the actual probability value and the nature of the significance test.	☐	☐	☐
✔ Present appropriate interpretations (e.g., NS, no effect; $P < .05$, proof).	☐	☐	☐
✔ Present the appropriate emphasis in displaying and interpreting the statistical analysis, in particular controlling for unplanned comparisons.	☐	☐	☐

Reprinted with permission from The Standards of Reporting Trials Group. A proposal for structured reporting of randomized controlled trials. *JAMA* 1994;272:1926–1931. Copyright 1994, American Medical Association.

*If the data analyst is not masked as to the interventions, new treatments may be grossly favored over standard treatments.[a]

†This information may show duplicate publication rather than two separate trials by the same author or group.

‡Many trials are longitudinal and require several follow-up assessments. These assessments may be subjective based on the questionnaire or scale responses. There is wide variation in how scales and questionnaires are constructed,[b] which may influence the assessment, reliability, validity, and responsiveness of the treatment outcome of interest. Providing information or references about the development of these outcome measures permits readers to judge how confident they should be about the results.

References

[a]Schulz KF, Chalmers I, Grimes DA, Altman DG. Assessing the quality of randomization from reports of controlled trials published in obstetrical and gynecology journals. *JAMA* 1994;272:125–128; and Gøtzsche PC. Bias in double-blind trials. *Dan Med Bull* 1990;37:329–336.

[b]McDowell I, Newell C. Measuring health: A guide to rating scales and questionnaires. New York: Oxford University Press, 1987; and Steiner DL, Norman DR. Health measurement scales: A practical guide to their development and use. Oxford, England: Oxford University Press, 1989.

Cross-sectional studies (also called "synchronic studies") provide a snapshot of the problem at a specific point in time. They also are called "prevalence studies" because only people with the specific disease or condition under study at the time of the snapshot are considered diseased. Cross-sectional studies make all measurements on a single occasion. A survey is an example of a cross-sectional study.

Example 3–10.

On a given day, researchers might measure the body temperature and presence of pressure ulcers in 100 patients in a nursing home.

Obviously, cross-sectional studies are not strong designs for proving causation because they measure risk factors and disease concurrently; however, they are comparatively easy, fast, and economical.

Before you begin a cross-sectional study, plan how you will document whether exposure to the study factor preceded the effect or disease. Fixed characteristics, such as height, race, and sex, must be analyzed separately from unfixed characteristics, such as weight, marital status, and blood pressure, so be sure to word your questions appropriately.

Example 3–11.

People often stop exercising when a disease develops. In a cross-sectional study, this lack of exercise could be misinterpreted as a risk factor for the disease.

In summary, you can classify most studies by answering two questions:

1. Were the events under study (exposure or treatment) changed as part of the study? If they were, the study was experimental. If they were not, the study was observational.
2. Were the measurements in this study made on more than one occasion? If not, the study was cross-sectional.

After you answer these two questions and understand this basic terminology, you can move on to planning the finer points of the study design.

CHAPTER 4.

Minimizing Bias

PRINCIPLE 19. PLAN TO MINIMIZE BIAS.

Bias is a "systematic error introduced into sampling or testing by selecting or encouraging one outcome or answer over others" (*Merriam-Webster's Collegiate Dictionary,* 1993). All studies contain random errors that are determined by chance. When errors are not determined by chance alone and produce results that depart **systematically** from true values, bias exists. Bias cannot be ignored.

Bias reduces the representativeness of the sample studied. A biased sample is a common problem in study designs and often is responsible for the rejection of manuscripts. During the planning phase, be careful to develop an unbiased protocol. The three main types of bias are:

1. Selection bias
2. Response bias
3. Information bias

Selection bias is a systematic difference between people who are selected for a study and those who are not selected. This type of bias is both common and lethal to your chances of publication. Selection bias can be caused by patient referral patterns, survival differences, or loss to follow-up.

To minimize selection bias in cohort studies, devise a strategy that will allow you to choose a random sample from a stable population and obtain adequate follow-up. A stable population is one in which you are able to obtain complete and accurate follow-up information on all or most members. To minimize selection bias you should strive to identify a group of people who plan to live in the same area for a long period and who are willing and able to cooperate with follow-up investigators.

What is an adequate follow-up period? The answer depends on the topic, but if you can show a longer follow-up period than the landmark papers, you will certainly improve the odds of publication. Develop a plan to obtain follow-up information for the entire sample, or at least a large percentage.

To some extent, you can control for the effect of selection bias statistically if you have variables to measure its direction and effect. For example, you can record why patients were lost to follow-up and the exact cause of death. In other situations, you can document why people did not participate in the study.

Response bias is a specific type of selection bias in which respondents differ systematically from nonrespondents.

Example 4–1.

People with a certain disease may be more likely to respond to a mailed questionnaire about the disease than people who are unaffected by the disease.

Information, or measurement, bias is a systematic difference between the measurements recorded in different study groups. In cohort studies, patients with a risk factor may be tested for the outcome more frequently and carefully than those without the risk factor. This situation is a special type of information bias called "surveillance" bias or "diagnostic suspicion" bias.

Recall bias, another type of information bias, occurs when people with a certain condition are more likely to "remember" exposure to the variable under study than people without the condition.

Example 4–2.

Parents of children with cancer may remember more information and provide greater detail about exposure to potentially carcinogenic factors than parents of children without cancer, even if both groups had identical exposure levels.

This situation can easily occur in case-control or cross-sectional studies, but not in cohort studies. In cohort studies, no one knows in which people the disease will develop in the future. Therefore, it is highly unlikely that these people can report a different level of exposure.

Other forms of bias include the following:

Confounding bias is the effect of extraneous variables that must be adjusted for, before the research question can be answered. Confounding variables are the variables that may account for the association between exposure and disease. Sometimes they mask the true association.

Example 4–3.

An inner-city hospital may have a higher neonatal mortality rate than the national average. Although the difference between these crude (unadjusted) mortality rates may be statistically significant, interpreting this difference as an indication of poor obstetric care probably would be incorrect. The confounding variables associated with inner-city life probably create a confounding bias. These factors must be adjusted for, before valid conclusions can be drawn.

In clinical research studies, selection bias, particularly attrition bias, is a common problem. *Attrition* is a reduction in the number of patients who remain in a study. Attrition bias occurs when the patients who drop out of a study are systematically different from those who complete the study.

Berkson's bias is a clinical selection bias that occurs when the rate of hospitalization differs between the cases and the controls. Patients with two overlapping conditions often are more likely to be admitted to the hospital. Researchers then may make the mistake of assuming an association between the two conditions if they analyze only the patients who are admitted to the hospital.

Prevalence/incidence (Neyman's) bias is caused by risk factors that prolong the disease, not cause it.

Table 4–1. Bias Reported by Reviewers and Editors
Sampling bias
Ascertainment bias (a measurement problem that can often be avoided by "blinding" the outcome measurement)
Data collection bias
Publication bias toward "positive" results (Studies with positive results are more likely to be published, leading to problems with meta-analysis interpretation; many researchers are reluctant to pursue and publish "negative" results.)
Reviewer bias (against an unknown author from a "minor" institution)
Self-promotion or agency promotion bias
Uncontrolled variables bias

Table 4–1 shows additional forms of bias reported by reviewers and editors.

Failure to recognize and control for these and other forms of bias is a classic mistake that clinicians make when analyzing medical research data.

Bias is a complex subject, but the main points to remember are as follows:

Plan to reduce bias to a minimum. If bias occurs, try to measure its effect so you can adjust for it statistically in your analysis. Document your efforts to reduce bias. During the planning phase, you can strengthen your study design by researching the specific types of bias and epidemiologic methods important for your particular study design and topic. Learn from previous researchers, and customize your study design to reduce bias.

⊕ FOR MORE INFORMATION

See Fleiss (1981); Fletcher, Fletcher, and Wagner (1996); Friedman (1994); Hulley and Cummings (1988); Last (1995); Mausner and Kramer (1985); Morton and Hebel (1990); Rothman (1986); Sackett (1979); Sackett et al. (1991).

CHAPTER 5.

The Data Collection Form

DESIGNING THE FORM

PRINCIPLE 20. Design a short, but comprehensive data collection form.

A common mistake that clinical researchers make is not investing enough time in creating a quality data collection form. Whether this form is a questionnaire for patients or a chart abstracting form for a research nurse, devoting ample resources to its creation enables one to avoid common mistakes and costly problems. The following principles related to questionnaires also can be used to improve most data collection forms.

Start with your most important questions, and focus on solving your principal research problem. Then decide how many variables you can include. Short questionnaires may have higher response rates than long ones, but a questionnaire that is too short may not solve the research problem at all. Always number each question. **Use questions with defined choices rather than open-ended questions.**

As you design the data collection form, write a coding guide to explain how to use the form. For example, explain how many decimal places to use, what units to use, and whether measurements should be recorded in metric units or the United States equivalent.

Ensure that the choices for each question cover all possibilities. Include questions to verify inclusion and exclusion criteria. Line up the choices vertically, and include the code with each choice on the data collection form to simplify data entry.

Example 5–1.

1. Race	1 ☐ White
	2 ☐ African-American
	3 ☐ Hispanic
	4 ☐ Asian
	9 ☐ Multiracial or other, specify
2. _____ ?	0 ☐ No 1 ☐ Yes
3. _____ ?	0 ☐ No 1 ☐ Yes
4. _____ ?	0 ☐ Disagree 1 ☐ Agree
5. _____ ?	Never Always 0 1 2 3 4 5

Note that in Example 5–1, for race, "multiracial or other" is coded as 9 to allow more categories to be added (5–8) during a study.

Choices should increase in value from left to right, as in question 5 in Example 5–1. Ask an experienced biostatistician to critique your questionnaire before you administer it. A biostatistician can identify and solve problems you may not notice, such as questions that instruct the respondent to check all answers that apply.

⊕ FOR MORE INFORMATION

Spilker and Schoenfelder (1991) provide several hundred examples in their book *Data Collection Forms in Clinical Trials*.

PRINCIPLE 21. UNDERSTAND HOW YOUR SAMPLE DIFFERS FROM THE LARGER POPULATION.

Especially for surveys and mailed questionnaires, decide how you will compare respondents with nonrespondents. You may have basic information from a mailing list about the respondents, such as age and sex. Or, you may be able to compare your respondents with published samples.

A different approach is to compare early respondents with late respondents. Nonrespondents tend to be similar to late respondents (Babbie 1990). To make this comparison, you must record the mailing date and the date of receipt for each survey. The information that you obtain from this comparison will allow you to assess the type and direction of response bias.

PRINCIPLE 22. CONDUCT A THOROUGH PILOT TEST OF YOUR QUESTIONNAIRE.

Use a pilot test on an available small group similar to your sample to determine whether the wording of the directions or of specific questions is confusing. Use a system of logical choices that makes sense to your sample. For example, educators may find letter grades (A–F) easier to use than numbers. However, remember that most answers are converted to numbers for data entry.

Including too many questions or too many of a certain type, such as open-ended questions, is an obvious problem. For the most part, omit repetitive questions, although to assess the consistency of a respondent's answers, some researchers repeat one or more questions, usually strategically separated from each other.

Delete or revise questions that most respondents in your pilot test did not understand. Make abstract questions concrete by including straightforward, neutral examples respondents can evaluate. During the pilot test, determine whether the respondents thought that some questions were asked merely for effect, with no answer expected. Delete these rhetorical questions; respondents will be annoyed that you wasted their time with these questions. Do not ask questions that lead the respondent toward a particular choice. If, in the pilot test, most people circled one choice, such as "occasionally," convert to more specific choices in the final version (e.g., "once a day," "once a week," "once a month").

From a statistical point of view, you ordinarily would want the answers to any one question to form a "normal" bell-shaped curve (distribution) on a frequency histogram. This distribution allows you to use a full range of statistical tools. So use the results of your pilot

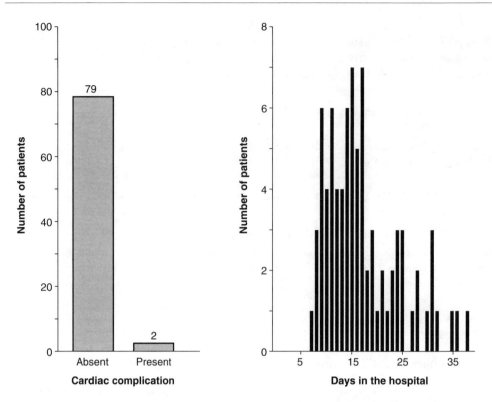

Figure 5–1. Graphs showing the differences between a *categorical* variable (left) and a *continuous* variable (right).

test to assess the extent to which your statistical analysis will be feasible. If not, perhaps you can include additional questions to make the analysis possible. As the example in Figure 5–1 demonstrates, outcome expressed as a continuous variable is often superior to outcome expressed categorically.

Including "dummy" questions can reduce various forms of bias, but only if respondents do not know the main risk factor or outcome you are testing. For example, if you are conducting a survey about alcohol use, you also can include questions about smoking, exercise, and eating habits.

Before you administer your questionnaire, try to solve the potentially devastating problems of respondents selecting more than one answer or not answering a question at all. Develop clear guidelines for defining invalid questionnaires that will be excluded from the analysis. For example, you might decide that at least 80% of the questions must be answered for a questionnaire to be considered valid.

If you spend adequate time creating, testing, and revising your questionnaire, your paper will have a much better chance of being published. Many investigators do not allow enough time or resources to develop a quality questionnaire. Always consult a colleague who has successfully designed questionnaires.

⊚ VITAL POINT

Quality questionnaires equal quality data.

⊕ FOR MORE INFORMATION

See Appendixes B and C for examples with solutions to many of these data collection form problems.

PRINCIPLE 23. IMPROVE YOUR RESPONSE RATE.

The success of a study that is based on a mailed questionnaire often depends on obtaining **a satisfactory response rate** (Figures 5–2 and 5–3). To improve your response rate for mailed questionnaires, consider the ideas shown in Tables 5–1 and 5–2.

⊕ FOR MORE INFORMATION

See the American Marketing Association's book, *Handbook for Customer Satisfaction* (see NTC Business Books in Appendix D) or Chapter 5 of Hulley and Cummings (1988) for more details about questionnaire design.

Mailing your questionnaire is not the only option. For example, you can administer them during mandatory employee training sessions. If you use this approach, ensure employee confidentiality and recruit someone whom the respondents trust to ask for their cooperation. This administration method improves the response rate to as high as 98%.

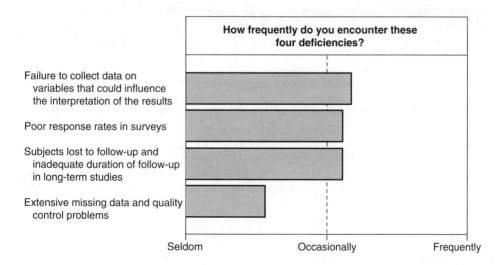

Figure 5–2. Frequency of problems with data quality. From question 25 of the Peer Review Questionnaire in Appendix B.

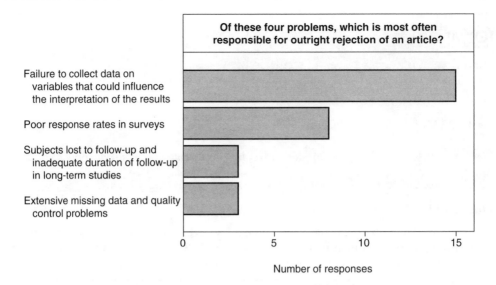

Figure 5–3. Data quality problems that result in rejection. From question 26 of the Peer Review Questionnaire in Appendix B.

Table 5–1.   Elements to Include in the Cover Letter of a Questionnaire
✔ The respondent's name in the salutation
✔ Relevance of the topic to the respondent
✔ Answers to questions that arose during the pilot study
✔ An explanation of your intentions
✔ An explanation of who is paying for the study (University sponsorship is better than corporate sponsorship [Fox, Crask, and Kim 1988].)
✔ An incentive for responding, but not $1. (A report of the findings may be a better incentive than a small sum.)
✔ The deadline for responding
✔ An estimate of the time needed to complete the questionnaire
✔ A postscript asking for cooperation

PRINCIPLE 24. TEST FOR RELIABILITY AND VALIDITY.

While reliability and validity of your measurements are important in clinical research, they are essential in questionnaire research.

Reliability (or precision) assesses consistency of measurement. Reliability is the degree to which an investigator can depend on a measuring instrument. When reliability is high, a test that is repeated on the same patient and under the same conditions will yield the same result.

Example 5–2.

A low-reliability variable is self-reported duration of exposure to passive smoke among women who are breastfeeding their infants. A high-reliability variable is the cotinine concentration in the mothers' breast milk.

Table 5–2.   Suggestions for Improving the Response Rate

- ✔ Print the questionnaire on green paper. Research suggests that questionnaires printed on green paper have a higher response rate (Fox, Crask, and Kim 1988). Any color that stands out from the white paper on most desks probably will improve the response rate. Avoid colors that make the survey difficult to read or appear unprofessional.
- ✔ For lengthy questionnaires or those on a sensitive topic, send a prenotification postcard or letter explaining that a questionnaire will arrive soon (Fox, Crask, and Kim 1988).
- ✔ Find a special third-party contact, ideally someone respected by the respondents (e.g., a union leader, society president). This contact person can ask the group for cooperation in completing and returning the surveys. A manager or supervisor may not be the ideal contact person, and may have a negative effect by creating a bias; you do not want subjects to feel pressured into completing the questionnaire. An article in a newsletter from an organization to which the respondents belong also may be helpful.
- ✔ Allow the respondents to express their concerns and make suggestions.
- ✔ Use first-class postage; bulk-rate postage suggests junk mail.
- ✔ Use stamps rather than metered mail; pay for return postage, but avoid business reply postage.
- ✔ For small surveys, consider using handwritten addresses.
- ✔ Send a follow-up survey in 2 to 3 weeks; you can often double your response rate with a second mailing.
- ✔ Five to six weeks after your initial mailing, send a postcard thanking respondents who have replied and a reminder to those who have not responded.

Inter-rater reliability measures how well different data collectors obtain the same information. In studies that have more than one person abstracting information from hospital charts, reporting your inter-rater reliability is important to the credibility of your conclusions.

Intra-rater reliability measures how well a person records the same information a second time. This factor is evaluated with the kappa, weighted kappa, and intraclass correlation tests. Consult an experienced statistician if you are not familiar with these statistics.

When you evaluate studies performed by others, do not simply accept a statement that reliability testing was done. Look carefully to determine whether the fundamental variables were tested for reliability. A good study provides sufficient information to permit evaluation of its reliability. Many inexperienced researchers have trouble assessing the reliability of their own research and critically evaluating reliability in published reports.

Validity is an index of how well a test or procedure measured what it is intended to measure.

Example 5–3.

Malnutrition could be assessed by asking patients to score their nutritional intake on a scale of 1 to 10, but measuring each patient's serum albumin level would have more validity.

During the planning phase, consider whether your questionnaire or data collection form is valid in comparison with other measures previously tested and published. When you write your paper, you may have to include the questions, or at least a sample of your wording, in your manuscript (or an appendix). You may also have to explain why you chose to use a new instrument rather than an existing instrument.

Internal validity is how accurately your conclusions described what actually occurred in the study.

Example 5–4.

Patients are interviewed about their daily alcohol consumption, but some respondents, probably the heavy drinkers, may not provide accurate answers.

External validity is the generalizability of your study, or the appropriateness of your conclusions to larger populations represented by your sample. A generalization is a broadly applicable statement, law, or principle derived from specifics.

Example 5–5.

A database of trauma patients pooled from major trauma centers around the country may be weighted toward poor inner-city patients. In a study that uses this database, conclusions about priorities for injury prevention may not be valid for suburban or rural populations. This study has a problem with external validity.

⊕ FOR MORE INFORMATION

See Rothman (1986).

CHAPTER 6.

Eligibility

PRINCIPLE 25. SELECT A GROUP OF PATIENTS THAT IS AS HOMOGENEOUS AS POSSIBLE.

Your research conclusions will be stronger if you study a group of patients with unilateral, simple, or isolated injuries. Do not make the common mistake of including a mixture of diseases or procedures. Do not add dissimilar types of subjects simply to increase the sample size.

Improper selection of patients reduces validity. To avoid this problem, define your inclusion criteria early in the planning phase. With the help of your colleagues, refine your definition until it is impossible to misunderstand or misconstrue. Ask yourself: "Could my colleagues obtain a similar sample by following my written instructions?" When the answer is "yes," you have completed an important part of the methods. Formalizing this definition of inclusion will prevent many problems during the study.

PRINCIPLE 26. BE CAREFUL IF YOU USE A "MIXED" SAMPLE.

Inclusion and exclusion decisions should be made by the entire research team, and only after careful consideration of the statistical and clinical implications. Careless exclusion decisions can quickly destroy a study. For studies with many criteria, consider creating a table of inclusion and exclusion criteria. For a good example, see Ewigman et al. (1993). If you included conditions that may raise eyebrows, plan to describe them in the Methods and Results sections.

 VITAL POINT

Including different conditions and disease states in the same study requires careful consideration regarding what conclusions can be drawn.

Some studies must include patients with different severities of a disease or complexities of a procedure. For this type of study, be prepared to explain your rationale. Specifically, clarify why patients with less severe conditions should be included in the study. Describe the distribution of the disease severity, and explain why you are studying patients across this distribution. Plan a method to show that you have statistically adjusted for differences among these patients. In small clinical studies, a dilemma occurs when the number of subjects with a specific poor outcome is too small to permit reasonable statistical analysis. Trying to solve this problem by combining different types of poor outcome leads to the following types of reviewer criticism:

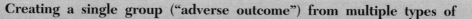

Lumping many adverse outcomes under one end point obscures the true relation between the tests and the individual end points. Apparently, the authors found this necessary because of the relatively small number of cases.

Creating a single group ("adverse outcome") from multiple types of

adverse outcomes is concerning. These outcomes are unlikely to have a single common source.

Remember, be careful when your dependent (outcome) variable includes several diverse conditions. If combining many adverse outcomes into one category is necessary, anticipate criticism. Include only those that are potentially predictable by the independent variables in the study. Provide data, justification, and references for each type of outcome. Explain your rationale for including each different outcome in the dependent variable. Provide results for both the individual types of adverse outcomes and the combined group. In your final draft, describe, discuss, and compare with the literature both ways of looking at this problem (combined and separated).

When you evaluate screening tests, your analysis will be more convincing if it is limited to one specific outcome, especially one that is biologically plausible to predict from such a screening test (Sackett et al. 1991).

PRINCIPLE 27. USE A REPRODUCIBLE METHOD TO DEFINE YOUR STUDY SUBJECTS.

After you define your sample, the next step is to verify that your criteria are not subjective. When you define the inclusion and exclusion criteria for the final analysis, use a method that is clearly objective. Verify that this definition is consistent throughout the manuscript.

For the definition of a disease, the International Classification of Diseases (ICD) codes are a good place to start. Verify that the codes include and exclude precisely what you intended. For the definition of a procedure, Current Procedural Terminology (CPT) codes provide more detail.

All diagnoses and procedures must be encoded for optimal computerized analysis. In question 45 of the data collection form in Appendix C, notice how multiple diagnoses are recorded with ICD codes. In the analysis phase, an unlimited number of variables can be created by defining ranges of codes.

Example 6–1.

By storing diagnoses in a computer using ICD codes, you can create a new variable called "HIPFX" for hip fractures by instructing the computer to look for the ICD codes from 820.00 through 820.99 in the diagnosis fields. A broader variable for all fractures could be computed with the ICD codes from 800.00 to 829.99.

You also can create a checklist for major groups of diagnoses. Checklists are useful when the ICD coding system does not provide enough detail for your project.

Three valuable coding references for clinical researchers are:

1. *St. Anthony's Illustrated Color-Coded ICD Code Book*
2. The *AMA CPT Code Book*
3. *St. Anthony's DRG Working Guidebook*

⊕ FOR MORE INFORMATION

See St. Anthony's Publishing or the American Medical Association in Appendix D.

CHAPTER 7.

Randomization, "Blinding," and Confidentiality

RANDOMIZATION AND BLINDING

PRINCIPLE 28. USE RANDOMIZATION AND "BLINDING" TO STRENGTHEN THE STUDY DESIGN AND MINIMIZE BIAS.

Whenever it is ethical and practical, consider using a randomized design. With random allocation, chance determines the assignment of subjects to study groups. To randomize subjects, most researchers use random number tables, which can be customized for your study with software programs such as True Epistat (see Appendix D). If you use a randomized design, follow all of the rules of randomization, and document your work.

The study design in which patients are randomly assigned to either receive or not receive the intervention under study is called a "randomized clinical trial." This type of study design is particularly strong because it permits researchers to assess whether the intervention is related to the outcome of interest by reducing the effect of other factors.

During the planning phase of your study, decide how you will use randomization. Some researchers believe that the methods of randomization are standardized, but this is not true. Many clinical research projects can be significantly improved with new and creative randomization strategies.

Blinding, which refers to keeping participants unaware of the treatment being given, also deserves sufficient planning. With a double-blinded design, clinicians are unaware of which patients receive the active treatment and which receive the placebo. With a triple-blinded design, which is useful for the interim analysis, the statistician (or in some cases, the person measuring the outcome) is unaware of which group received active treatment. For obvious reasons, ophthalmologists often prefer to use the term "masked" rather than "blinded."

For clinical trials, document the elements of treatment in detail and describe your motivation for comparing these factors. You should have a theoretical model driving your project. So record in your research notes the rationale for each element of treatment. For all randomized controlled trials, be prepared to report all of the items shown in Table 3–2. Remember, randomization also can strengthen many other research designs, such as mailed questionnaires and even chart reviews.

Example 7–1.

A study is being planned in which four research nurses will review the hospital charts of trauma patients who were admitted to 10 hospitals. Investigators who are planning the study design are concerned about problems with inter-rater reliability. They know from a pilot study that two of the research nurses are much more aggressive in searching the charts for complications. To minimize this potential bias, they use a random number table to assign monthly blocks of charts to be reviewed at the 10 hospitals by the four research nurses. Although this study is not a randomized clinical trial, the use of randomization strengthens the study design and reduces bias.

CONFIDENTIALITY

PRINCIPLE 29. PROTECT THE CONFIDENTIALITY OF ALL PARTICIPANTS.

Institutional Review Board (IRB) approval and informed consent are important parts of the modern research design. Even when you think that IRB approval may not be required, budget sufficient time for this review early in your project. A major element of IRB approval is confidentiality. Protecting patient, hospital, and physician confidentiality not only is ethical, but also protects you from lawsuits and generally is a requirement for publication.

In your research database, use sequential "case numbers" (i.e., 1, 2, 3 . . .) for patients, hospitals, and physicians. Using case numbers instead of names protects patient confidentiality, which is especially important in studies that involve HIV or other sensitive subjects. The principal investigator should keep a notebook matching names and case numbers in a locked file cabinet along with the research files and backup diskettes.

If you plan to publish tables that list patients, use sequential case numbers, not patient names or initials. When investigators do not adequately address confidentiality, reviewers may ask:

Were anonymity and confidentiality assured to your subjects?

Be prepared to explain in the Methods section of your manuscript what steps you took to protect confidentiality and whether IRB approval was obtained. Documentation of IRB approval may be a requirement of publication, so be prepared.

FOR MORE INFORMATION

See Hulley and Cummings (1988) or the Food and Drug Administration (FDA) Internet Web site (see Appendix D). The FDA provides information sheets, such as "An Informed Consent and the Clinical Investigator" and "A Guide to Informed Consent Documents." Also refer to the Declaration of Helsinki (World Medical Association 1997, and Appendix E), the Federal Register (Protection of Human Subjects 1991), and the Guidelines on Structure and Content of Clinical Study Reports (International Conference on Harmonisation 1996).

CHAPTER 8.

End Points and Outcome

UNIT OF ANALYSIS

PRINCIPLE 30. CHOOSE THE OPTIMAL UNIT OF ANALYSIS BEFORE YOU BEGIN TO COLLECT DATA.

The unit of analysis usually is an individual patient, but not always. For some studies, it is a hospital, a population of residents of a particular country, or even a breast with one or more implants.

Example 8–1.

A group of investigators is planning a study of pregnant women to evaluate the accuracy of screening for fetal problems. The group must answer several questions: How should twins be analyzed? How should a woman who has two deliveries during the study period be analyzed? Should abortions and stillbirths be excluded? Should the unit of analysis be: (1) a pregnant woman; (2) an infant; (3) a pregnancy; or (4) a singleton (one fetus) pregnancy that continues beyond 28 weeks of gestation?

To choose an appropriate unit of analysis, you must think through the intended data analysis. **You can save time and money by consulting a statistician, particularly one who is willing to invest the time to learn your research subject thoroughly.**

⊚ VITAL POINT

You must decide on the unit of analysis before you collect any data.

CONFOUNDING FACTORS

PRINCIPLE 31. ANTICIPATE CONFOUNDING FACTORS.

Confounding factors, or *confounders,* are all of the "other things" that could explain your results. They are predictor variables that **must** be controlled, before you can truly analyze your data.

Confounding factors are extraneous variables that distort the apparent association between exposure and disease or distort the size of the effect of a study factor. When investigators do not adjust for important confounding factors, their results must be interpreted carefully.

Crude rates are statistics not adjusted for confounding factors. Crude rates are calculated as the number of events in a population over time. They are tabulated without being broken down into classes.

"*Adjusted rates* are summary statistics that have undergone statistical transformation to permit fair comparison between groups differing in some characteristic that may affect risk of disease" (Mausner and Kramer 1985).

Case mix, or *patient mix,* refers to baseline differences (in severity of illness or injury, preexisting conditions, or the characteristics of patients) among a group of patients.

Example 8–2.

If an investigator wants to compare survival rates among hospitals for patients who underwent a specific surgical procedure, crude survival rates are almost meaningless. The investigator must adjust for confounding factors, such as differences in the patients (e.g., age), preexisting conditions (e.g., diabetes), and whether the procedure was performed on an emergency or an elective basis. Collectively, these factors are referred to as "case mix" or "patient mix."

◎ VITAL POINT

Before you collect any data, develop a strategy to control for as many confounding factors as possible, especially those that could affect the outcome of interest.

Perform a literature search to identify other variables that may be correlated with your outcome. Record these variables so that you can confirm or refute these reports through your analysis. You may decide to reproduce the tables and figures from landmark papers with your data.

Recording potential confounding factors, such as smoking history, during data collection saves time and money. If you overlook an important confounding factor, you may have to search for the information later. This search not only wastes time, but also may produce poor-quality data.

Identify several strategies to control for confounding factors, and anticipate the problems associated with each strategy. Choose the strongest design that fits your budget and schedule. Document your strategy, and cite a reference to support it. Ignoring this step may lead to the following comments from reviewers:

 This study is interesting in concept, but flawed in execution.

 I would suspect that X was a major factor, although it is difficult to determine this from such a crude assessment as Y levels. It would have been better to have presented mean daily or monthly Z values.

CLASSIFICATION OF VARIABLES

PRINCIPLE 32. DISTINGUISH BETWEEN INDEPENDENT AND DEPENDENT VARIABLES.

Independent, or input, variables ordinarily have values that are autonomous of the dependent, or outcome, variables (Figure 8–1). Usually, independent variables are graphed on the X-axis (horizontal axis). Because independent variables precede dependent variables, they often are called "predictors." In epidemiology, independent variables are called "risk factors" or "exposure variables." Remember, independent variables are antecedents; dependent variables are consequents.

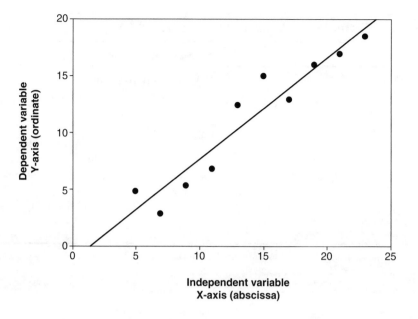

Figure 8–1. Independent and dependent variables.

Dependent, or output, variables have responses that are contingent on independent variables. They usually are graphed on the Y-axis (vertical axis) and often are called "outcome variables."

Example 8–3.

In a study to identify patients at high risk for pneumonia, pneumonia is the outcome, or dependent, variable. To predict this outcome, the investigator can analyze age, sex, and smoking history. These are the independent variables. During the analysis, the investigator might decide to control for age and determine whether sex is a significant predictor of pneumonia—independent of age. In this case, age is treated as a confounding factor that is adjusted for, statistically.

PRINCIPLE 33. RECORD OUTCOME WITH SEVERAL VARIABLES.

Whenever possible, identify several variables that you can use to measure short-term and long-term outcome in your study. If you have technical problems with one dependent variable, you may be able to use another variable to answer the research question.

When your success rests on one dependent variable, choose the strongest possible variable. The ideal dependent variable is reproducible, objective, and standardized. It is measured as a continuous variable and has a frequency histogram with a normal bell-shaped curve.

Continuous variables are measurements (e.g., hematocrit). *Categorical variables* are labels for groups (e.g., anemia). *Dichotomous variables* are categorical variables with only two groups, such as alive versus dead. For dichotomous dependent variables, the statistically ideal situation is to have 50% of patients with each outcome.

Table 8–1. Examples of Weak and Strong Variables	
Weak	*Strong*
DRG outlier	Days hospitalized beyond the DRG limit
Anemic	Hematocrit or hemoglobin level
Low birth weight	Exact birth weight
Respiratory distress syndrome	Lung index
Hypertensive	Maximum or average daily systolic, diastolic, and mean blood pressure from ambulatory monitoring, or trough-to-peak ratios
NICU admission°	Total cost of hospitalization or days in the NICU

° Admission to the neonatal intensive care unit (NICU) is a weak variable because it includes many infants who are admitted for 1 day of observation.

To improve the value of your dependent variable, avoid using variables that are uniform or nearly uniform for all patients. For example, in a study in which the mortality rate is extremely low, a more useful outcome variable may be the morbidity rate or number of days in the hospital (see Figure 5–1). For continuous dependent variables, you can recode and combine the results into a categorical variable, such as less than versus greater than or equal to the median value. Table 8–1 shows examples of weak and strong dependent variables.

Example 8–4.

Length of stay in the hospital is often a skewed continuous dependent variable. Creating a new variable that is set to 0 for patients whose stay is less than the median and set to 1 for the other patients will produce two even groups of patients to analyze. Even if the sample is small, this approach allows the use of many powerful statistical techniques.

Ask yourself: "How could reviewers see my dependent variable as inadequate or problematic?" Include additional dependent variables to control for these problems. Also consider the patient's perspective. For example, does your dependent variable measure success in the same way that patients define success?

⊕ FOR MORE INFORMATION

Before you begin to collect data, you may want to research the current methods of assessing quality-of-life outcomes. See Testa and Simonson (1996) and the six articles on the quality of care that were published in the *New England Journal of Medicine* in 1996 (Angell and Kassirer 1996; Berwick 1996; Blumenthal 1996 part I and part IV; Blumenthal and Epstein 1996; Brook et al. 1996; Chassin 1996). These articles and others have been compiled in the book *Quality of Care* (The New England Journal of Medicine 1997). For randomized clinical trials, see Chapter 15 of the book by Bulpitt (1996).

PREPARING FOR DATA ENTRY

PRINCIPLE 34. QUANTIFY, QUANTIFY, QUANTIFY!

You can simplify data analysis by addressing some important points during the planning phase. First, choose variables that can be quantified and will thereby provide the strongest statistical analysis. Then strive for ways to measure these variables more precisely.

Example 8–5.

If smoking is a central factor in your study, do not classify patients simply as smokers or nonsmokers. Quantify their smoking by including questions such as the following:

1. *Have you smoked at least 100 cigarettes in your entire life?**	0 ☐	*No*	
	1 ☐	*Yes*	
2. *Do you now smoke cigarettes:*	0 ☐	*Not at all*	
	1 ☐	*Some days*	
	2 ☐	*Every day*	
3. *How many cigarettes do you smoke each day?*	☐	☐	
4. *How many years have you been smoking?*	☐	☐	
5. *If you are a former smoker, how many years ago did you quit smoking?*	☐	☐	
6. *At what age did you begin smoking daily?*	☐	☐	

*Question 1 may appear odd, but it is a reproducible method of distinguishing people who "tried smoking" from those who were actual smokers.

Use an interval scale when possible. For certain variables, however, a checklist of **ordinal** choices (see Table 10–1) provides more accurate and complete data.

Example 8–6.

Many people are reluctant to disclose their exact annual income, but on a questionnaire, many respondents will check off an income range, such as < $10,000, $10,000–$20,000, and so forth. If you use this approach, make the categories meaningful by doing some homework. For example: What is the median income? What ranges will produce four income groups with even numbers of respondents? This investment in planning will pay off during data analysis.

Always use a pilot test to determine how to convert text answers into numeric categories. Remember, for statistical analysis that will draw out the truth from your numbers, you must quantify the exposure of the key variables.

Use a logical coding system, and avoid awkward conversions, such as the following:

$$1 = none, 2 = one, 3 = two$$
$$1 = second\ degree, 2 = third\ degree$$

For statistical analysis, the most effective coding is as follows:

$$0 = no, 1 = yes$$

Most variables should be coded as 0 and 1. Avoid mixing text and codes: provide a code for "other," and create a separate field for a text description of the "other" option. Create numeric codes for variables such as county, town, and race. Do not record data that cannot easily be analyzed with statistical software.

If you must use text, keep it short and uniform, such as the two-letter uppercase abbreviations for states used by the United States Postal Service. Avoid using embedded blanks in text. When an age is missing, use a code (e.g., -99) or leave the space blank. Do not enter text, such as NA or "Not Doc." Example 8–7 shows coding for computerized statistical analysis.

Example 8–7.

Problematic Format	Preferred Format
Restraint device used: [ ]	Was the occupant wearing a seat belt? 0 □ No 1 □ Yes 9 □ Unknown
Possible answers:	Possible answers:
SEAT BELT SEATBELT Seatbelt Unknown SB+Air Bag None NONE NA Not Doc (Blank)	0 1 9

Sample Size

ESTIMATING SAMPLE SIZE

PRINCIPLE 35. CONSIDER THE SAMPLE SIZE REQUIREMENTS OF YOUR RESEARCH EARLY IN THE PLANNING PHASE.

An important part of planning your study is choosing the size of the overall sample and subgroups. Many investigators have problems with analysis because they use small subgroups. Your overall sample may appear large, but when the findings are broken down into different types of patients and different types of treatment, your subgroups may be too small to provide meaningful information.

◎ VITAL POINT

Plan to study a large sample, with an adequate number in the control group and in important subgroups.

Calculating a sample size often requires judgments based on experience. For your first few studies, you may want to ask a statistician for help. A statistician can help you to estimate the size of your sample, design your data collection form, and analyze your data. An experienced statistician will tailor a plan for statistical analysis based on your specific data set. Avoid statisticians who use a template approach and do not consider the specific needs of your study. When you consult a statistician about the sample size needed, provide specific information about your study, such as the measurements used, the percentage of respondents in each group, the expected dropout rate, and how certain you must be in detecting a difference.

Consult with your research team and review sample sizes from similar published studies to determine whether your sample is too small to allow worthwhile conclusions to be drawn. If your sample is too small, enlarge it by collecting data on more patients, or refocus your study.

If you cannot collect your own data, consider using existing databases, such as trauma registries, hospital billing databases, and databases from your state health department. Secondary data analysis has limitations, however, and you may not have the precise variables or quality of data you need.

PRINCIPLE 36. CALCULATE THE SAMPLE SIZE REQUIRED TO DEFINITIVELY ADDRESS YOUR RESEARCH QUESTION.

Determine whether your sample size is adequate before you write your paper, and, ideally, before you collect any data. The following three methods are used to estimate sample sizes:

1. Tables
2. Formulas
3. Computer programs

Although sample size estimates are most useful during the planning phase, they also can shed light on your findings after the analysis and can provide valuable information for future research.

You can use a software program such as True Epistat to calculate sample sizes (see Appendix D), but remember, no method of calculating sample size is perfect. An experienced researcher (such as your chairman) can weigh the necessary information (e.g., cost, time required) to estimate the sample size. This perspective is often very valuable. In some cases, a small sample (or a low response rate) of high-quality information is preferable to a large sample of questionable data. For example, I included Nobel Prize winners in my survey for this book, even though it was obvious that most would not respond.

⊕ FOR MORE INFORMATION

Statistical Methods for Rates and Proportions by Fleiss (1981) provides excellent tables and formulas for estimating sample sizes. Also see Dawson-Saunders and Trapp (1994).

STATISTICAL POWER

To plan your study effectively, you must understand the concept of *statistical power*, which has been defined as:

1. "the probability of rejecting the null hypothesis where it is false" (*American Heritage Dictionary* 1996).
2. "the probability of rejecting the null hypothesis in a statistical test when a particular alternative hypothesis happens to be true" (*Merriam-Webster's Collegiate Dictionary* 1993).

Remember that P is the probability that a difference (or association) as large as the one you observed could have occurred by chance alone.

Example 9–1.

Suppose that drug A has a 50% success rate and drug B has a 25% success rate. If a study randomizes 65 patients into the drug A group and 65 patients into the drug B group, the investigator will have an 80% chance of detecting this difference and showing a statistically significant difference (P value of less than 0.05). The investigator also has a 20% chance of not detecting this difference and might incorrectly conclude that the success rates of these two drugs are similar. The power of this study is 80%.

Power is operationally defined as the probability that your study design will allow you to show a statistically significant difference between groups that are truly different. Power is equal to $1 -$ Beta. Beta is the probability of a type II error (see Principle 114). Larger studies usually have greater power. Table 9–1 shows sample size requirements. Example 9–2 shows how to use Table 9–1.

Example 9–2.

Suppose that you want to estimate the sample size that is necessary to determine whether a new antibiotic can improve the cure rate from 75% to 85% (assuming

Table 9–1. Sample Size Requirements for Each of Two Groups*,†

Group I	Group II																	
	5%	10%	15%	20%	25%	30%	35%	40%	45%	50%	55%	60%	65%	70%	75%	80%	85%	90%
10%	474																	
15%	160	725																
20%	88	219	945															
25%	58	113	270	1134														
30%	43	71	134	313	1291													
35%	33	50	82	151	348	1416												
40%	27	38	57	91	165	376	1511											
45%	22	30	42	62	98	175	395	1573										
50%	18	24	32	45	65	103	182	407	1605									
55%	16	20	26	34	47	68	106	186	411	1605								
60%	14	17	21	27	36	48	69	107	186	407	1573							
65%	12	14	18	22	28	36	49	69	106	182	395	1511						
70%	10	12	15	18	22	28	36	48	68	103	175	376	1416					
75%	9	11	13	15	18	22	28	36	47	65	98	165	348	1291				
80%	8	9	11	13	15	18	22	27	34	45	62	91	151	313	1134			
85%	7	8	9	11	13	15	18	21	26	32	42	57	82	134	270	945		
90%	6	7	8	9	11	12	14	17	20	24	30	38	50	71	113	219	725	
95%	5	6	7	8	9	10	12	14	16	18	22	27	33	43	58	88	160	474

These estimates use an alpha = 0.05 and a power = 0.80

* **How to use this table:** To find the sample size required to compare the proportions in two groups of equal size:
  1. Find the percentage in Group I in the left column.
  2. Find the percentage in Group II along the top row.
  3. If the percentage in Group II is greater than the percentage in Group I, reverse row and column in steps 1 and 2.
  4. The number at the intersection is the sample size required for each of the two groups.

† For details of the calculations and formulas used to compute the values in this table, see the original source. Data from Fleiss JL: *Statistical Methods for Rates and Proportions*, 2nd ed. New York, John Wiley, 1981, pp 260–280; and Fleiss JL, Tytun A, Ury HK: A simple approximation for calculating sample sizes for comparing independent proportions. *Biometrics* 36:343–346, 1980.

a power of 80% and a P value less than 0.05). Find 75% along the top row of Table 9–1. Then find 85% along the left column. These numbers intersect at the number 270, which means that you must include 270 patients in each of these two groups. If the difference actually is this large, you would have an 80% chance of detecting the difference and showing a P value of less than 0.05.

⊕ FOR MORE INFORMATION

See Chapter 13 of Hulley and Cummings (1988).

CHAPTER 10.

Preparing for Statistical Analysis

PLANNING THE ANALYSIS

PRINCIPLE 37. CONSIDER THE LEVEL OF MEASUREMENT FOR EACH OF YOUR VARIABLES.

To apply the appropriate statistical tests, you must understand the three basic levels of measurement (Table 10–1):

1. Nominal
2. Ordinal
3. Interval

Table 10–1. Levels of Measurement

Level	Explanation
Nominal (categorical variables)	Numbers are only labels for categories
Examples:	0 = no, 1 = yes 0 = nonsmoker, 1 = smoker 1 = white, 2 = black, 3 = Hispanic, 4 = Asian, 9 = other 1 = male, 2 = female
Note:	The categories can be numbered in any order without affecting the results: 1 = black, 2 = Hispanic, 3 = Asian, 4 = other, 9 = white 1 = female, 2 = male
Ordinal	Numbers are used to provide rank ordering (as in a horse race); these variables may be subjective
Examples:	1 = first, 2 = second, 3 = third 0–10 Apgar score 0 = nonsmoker, 1 = light smoker, 2 = moderate smoker, 3 = heavy smoker
Interval (continuous variables)	Numbers have equal intervals between successive points; this type of measurement typically is more objective than the other types
Examples:	Age Hematocrit Serum albumin level Cigarettes smoked per day

PRINCIPLE 38. ORGANIZE YOUR VARIABLES INTO CLINICALLY LOGICAL GROUPS.

Clearly distinguish between inclusion criteria variables, risk factors, and outcome variables. Be careful if using the same condition for more than one of these groups. The success of your statistical analysis may depend on how well you plan the collection and grouping of risk factors.

PRINCIPLE 39. DEMONSTRATE THAT THE STUDY GROUPS ARE COMPARABLE.

Use the same selection criteria for all treatment and control groups. Uniformity of treatment groups is a major concern of reviewers, as shown by the following comment:

> **Are patients in one group weighted in one direction? Do they have more severe or chronic problems? Is the average age different between the groups?**

PRINCIPLE 40. ESTABLISH A VALID CONTROL GROUP.

A *control group* is a set of subjects who are treated in the same way as a treatment group, absent the intervention being tested. The control group is the standard of comparison in judging experimental effects.

An absent or inappropriate control group is a major problem in many clinical studies. The entire research team should help to define the ideal control group and then critique it. Some studies benefit from the use of more than one control group. Reviewers will reject a well-written paper if they perceive that the control group is "a mishmash" or "too small." When you search the literature, study how various types of control groups are used for your particular topic.

⊕ FOR MORE INFORMATION

See Baker (1986), Bulpitt (1996), Friedman (1994), Hulley and Cummings (1988), Last (1995), Mausner and Kramer (1985), and Morton and Hebel (1990).

PLANNING THE FOLLOW-UP

PRINCIPLE 41. INCLUDE AN IMPRESSIVE LENGTH OF FOLLOW-UP.

When you plan a study, strive for a longer than average follow-up period. For some orthopedic journals, the required follow-up period is 2 years for most patients, 5 years for patients who undergo reconstructive procedures, and maturity for children. Consult clinical specialists from several disciplines to establish the optimal "window of follow-up" for each outcome.

For studies of long-term outcome performed in the United States, record each patient's name, date of birth, Social Security number, Medicare number, and (when they become available) universal patient identifier code. You can use the *National Death Index* (US Public Health Service 1981) to determine whether patients who were lost to follow-up by conventional methods have died. Since 1979, the National Center for

Health Statistics has maintained a database of all deaths in the United States (see Appendix D). You should also record the name, address, and telephone number of the patient's physician and the name, address, and telephone number of a friend or relative of the patient.

PRINCIPLE 42. CONSIDER THE IMPLICATIONS OF DIFFERENCES IN FOLLOW-UP TIME.

Establish a plan to analyze your data which addresses the possibility that the average follow-up time may differ between the treatment and control groups. Measure the range of time "at risk" for both groups. Consider excluding patients from the control group unless they have adequate time at risk. Control for time at risk in the analysis because it might be an important confounding variable.

Example 10–1.

Before an investigator can analyze the results of a study of occupational stress, the investigator must consider each participant's length of time at the job and the various types of bias that could affect the follow-up data.

Include in your study the number and percentage of patients who are lost to follow-up at the close of the study, and explain (in the Discussion section) how this number affects your results. If you plan to use survival analysis to adjust for follow-up differences, recognize the assumptions that must be met. One assumption is that the "censored" patients are similar to the uncensored patients. Resolve these problems during the planning phase of your study.

"Censored" is a term that is used to refer to a patient who was alive at the last contact with the researchers. For life-table analysis, this term is used to identify patients who have follow-up data to enter the particular interval, but whose most current follow-up data do not extend to the end of the interval. The number of patients withdrawn (who died) during this interval is used for survival analysis calculations.

Intention-to-treat (ITT) analysis includes data from all patients who were randomized into treatment or control groups, regardless of their compliance or the treatment they actually received. Analyzing only the patients who completed the study (actual on-therapy analysis, on-randomized treatment (ORT), or per protocol analysis) can create bias problems and seriously hinder your chance of publication in a high-quality journal.

⊕ **FOR MORE INFORMATION**

See Bulpitt (1996).

CHAPTER 11.

Avoiding Common Criticisms

PEER REVIEWERS' RESPONSES

PRINCIPLE 43. ANTICIPATE AND AVOID COMMON CRITICISMS.

Table 11–1 shows the answers that peer reviewers gave when they were asked to identify their most common criticisms of manuscripts.

Table 11–1. Reviewers' Most Common Criticisms of Manuscripts*

Design of the Study
- Poor experimental design
- Vague or inadequate description of methodology
- Biased data collection or inadequate sample
- No control or improper control
- Methodologic flaw
- No hypothesis
- Small sample size
- Nonrandom samples
- Statistically inadequate
- Univariate statistics when multivariate statistics were needed

Interpretation of the Findings
- Erroneous and unsupported conclusions
- Conclusions based on noncontrolled data
- Study design that does not support inferences
- Overinterpretation of data
- Inadequate link of findings to practice or policy
- Failure to consider alternative explanations of results
- Inadequate discussion

Importance of the Topic
- Rehash of established facts
- Insignificant research question
- Irrelevant or unimportant topic
- Low reader interest
- Little clinical relevance

(continued)

Table 11–1. Reviewers' Most Common Criticisms of Manuscripts* (*continued*)

Presentation of the Results

- Poorly focused
- Poorly organized
- Poorly written

*From question 1 of the Peer Review Questionnaire in Appendix B

Four major categories of criticism were identified by Kassirer and Campion (1994). Problems with study design are currently the most common problems (see Figure 3–1); be sure, during the planning stage, to identify and address these problems.

EDITORS' RESPONSES

Table 11–2 shows the responses of editors who were asked to report their most common criticisms of manuscripts.

Table 11–2. Editors' Most Common Criticisms of Manuscripts*

Design of the Study

- Inadequate study design
- Poor methodology, yielding potentially faulty results
- Failure to account for confounding factors
- Methods lacking sufficient rigor
- Biased protocol
- Lack of validity and reliability
- Inappropriate use of statistics
- Inappropriate comparisons
- Statistical methods not applied or used improperly
- Too few patients to permit meaningful conclusions

Interpretation of the Findings

- Unfounded conclusions
- Conclusions disproportionate to the results
- Uncritical acceptance of statistical results
- Improper inferences
- Unexplained inconsistencies

(continued)

Table 11–2.   Editors' Most Common Criticisms of Manuscripts* (continued)

- Failure to acknowledge methodologic flaws
- Inflation of the importance of the findings
- Interpretation of the results not concordant with the data

Importance of the Topic
- Lack of originality
- Insufficient new information
- Not generalizable
- Repetitious data (already in the literature or adding little)

Presentation of the Results
- Too long, verbose
- Excessively self-promotional
- Poor grammar, syntax, or spelling
- Somewhat anecdotal
- Poor organization
- Poorly written abstract
- Failure to communicate clearly

*From question 1 of the Peer Review Questionnaire in Appendix B

As with reviewers, editors were most concerned with study design. Editors also were concerned with the importance of the topic, whereas reviewers focused on the interpretation of the findings.

CHAPTER 12.

Preparing to Write a Publishable Paper

ORGANIZING YOUR MATERIAL INTO A MANUSCRIPT

PRINCIPLE 44. ORGANIZE YOUR INFORMATION INTO THE SECTIONS OF A MANUSCRIPT AS SOON AS POSSIBLE.

Before you collect any data, develop a clear plan for organizing your paper. Having such a plan will allow you to enter information into your word processing file efficiently. Medical manuscripts typically are arranged as shown in Table 12–1.

Table 12–1.   Order of Manuscript Sections with an Example of Page Limits

Manuscript Section	Pages
Cover letter	1
Copyright transfer page	1
Title page (numbered as page 1)	1
Condensation or précis (a summary of an article that usually is included with the table of contents), if required	1
Abstract and key words	1
Text	
Introduction	1
(Materials and) methods	4
Results	3
Discussion, with conclusions	2
Acknowledgments and support information	1
References	3
Tables, with titles and footnotes	3
Figure legends	1
Photocopy of each figure°	2
Total:	25

°Attach to each copy of the manuscript a set of glossy prints of the figures in a medium envelope.

CHOOSING A JOURNAL

PRINCIPLE 45. SELECT A TARGET JOURNAL BEFORE YOU BEGIN TO WRITE YOUR PAPER.

Plan to submit your paper to the journal most appropriate to the strength of your study and reader interest in your topic. The most prestigious journal in your field may not be the most appropriate for your paper. Although some researchers always send their manuscripts to a leading journal first, these journals usually have a low acceptance rate. On the other hand, they often provide excellent peer review comments.

In selecting a journal, consider the following factors:

- Reader interest
- Circulation
- Inclusion in *Index Medicus*
- Acceptance rate
- Publication lag
- Impact factor

Tables 12–2 through 12–5 provide information on circulation, impact factor, *Index Medicus* status, and acceptance rate for a selection of journals.

Publication lag is the interval between acceptance and publication; the average lag is 7 months.

⊕ FOR MORE INFORMATION

See "Summary Report of Journal Operations" in the annual archival issue of the *American Psychologist* (e.g., *Am Psychologist* 15:876–877, 1996).

The *impact factor* for a journal is defined as the number of times that articles from that journal have been cited during the previous 2 years divided by the total number of articles published by the journal during this period. To find a journal's impact factor, ask the

Table 12–2. Total Worldwide Circulation of Selection of Refereed Medical Journals (English Language Version, 1994–1995)

Journal	Approximate Circulation°	Impact Factor[†]	Index Medicus[‡]
JAMA (*Journal of the American Medical Association*)	372,000	6.863	Yes
RN (*Registered Nurse*)	285,000	NL	No
American Journal of Nursing	233,000	NL	Yes
New England Journal of Medicine	223,588	22.673	Yes
Emergency Medicine	167,000[§]	NL	No
Science	165,000	22.067	Yes
American Family Physician	150,000[§]	0.354	Yes
Consultant	129,800	NL	No
Postgraduate Medicine	125,889	0.277	Yes
Hospital Practice	115,000[§]	0.338	Yes
BMJ (*British Medical Journal*)	112,000[§]	4.411	Yes
Archives of Internal Medicine	100,000	4.137	Yes
Mayo Clinic Proceedings	95,588[‖]	1.814	Yes
Annals of Internal Medicine	95,000°	9.887	Yes
Critical Care Nurse	95,000[§]	NL	No
Hospital Physician (Internal and Family Medicine Edition)	90,000	NL	No
Nursing Times	87,348	NL	No
Journal of Respiratory Diseases	86,000	NL	No

(continued)

Table 12–2. Total Worldwide Circulation of Selection of Refereed Medical Journals (English Language Version, 1994–1995) (*continued*)

Journal	Approximate Circulation°	Impact Factor†	Index Medicus‡
Journal of Family Practice	76,000	0.904	Yes
American Journal of Critical Care	74,000	NL	Yes
Patient Outcomes	55,000	NL	No
Pediatrics	55,000§	2.840	Yes
Cleveland Clinic Journal of Medicine	54,000	0.279	Yes
American Journal of Medicine	53,751	2.703	Yes
AORN Journal	50,389	NL	Yes
American Board of Family Practice Journal	50,223	NL	No
Contemporary Surgery	50,000	NL	No
Cutis	49,000	0.317	Yes
Western Journal of Medicine	46,000	0.387	Yes
Humane Medicine	45,000	0.140	No
American Journal of Psychiatry	44,000	4.570	Yes
Lancet	40,000§	17.332	Yes
Clinical Diabetes	40,000	NL	No
Contemporary OB-GYN	39,255	NL	No
Anesthesiology	39,168	4.711	Yes
Archives of Surgery	39,000	2.402	Yes
Archives of General Psychiatry	38,500	11.416	Yes
Journal of Bone and Joint Surgery (American Volume)	38,260§	1.462	Yes
JAOA (Journal of the American Osteopathic Association)	38,000	NL	Yes
Radiology	35,684	3.800	Yes
Hospital Medicine	34,000	NL	No
Journal of Clinical Psychiatry	32,600°	3.130	Yes
Clinical Pediatrics	31,481	0.441	Yes
Journal of the American College of Cardiology	31,135°	6.013	Yes
Texas Medicine	31,000	NL	Yes
Southern Medical Journal	31,000	0.335	Yes
Nature	30,821	25.466	Yes
American Journal of Cardiology	30,500	2.253	Yes
Contemporary Orthopaedics	30,000	NL	No
Scientific American Medicine	30,000	NL	No

NL = not listed in the *Science Citation Index/Journal Citation Reports.*

° Source for circulation figures: *Ulrich's International Periodicals Directory.* 34th ed. New Providence (NJ): RR Bowker; 1996.

† Source for impact factor information: 1994 *Science Citation Index Journal Citation Reports.* Philadelphia: Institute for Scientific Information; 1995

‡ Source for Index Medicus status: *List of Journals Indexed in Index Medicus, 1996.* Washington (DC): National Library of Medicine; 1996.

§ Data provided by the journal editor or staff; figures are meant to reflect paid circulation, but some figures include unpaid circulation as well.

‖ Mayo Clinic Proceedings is sent free, on request, to physicians and third- and fourth-year medical students in the United States. Foreign subscribers and medical libraries pay a subscription fee.

Table 12–3. *Science Citation Index* Journal Citation Reports* Impact Factor for a Selection of Index Medicus† Journals (1994)

Journal	Impact Factor†	Approximate Circulation‡
Journal of Investigative Medicine	57.778	11,675
Annual Review of Biochemistry	42.169	NA
Annual Review of Immunology	39.426	NA
Cell	39.191	15,500
Annual Review of Cell and Developmental Biology	27.605	NA
Nature	25.466	30,821
New England Journal of Medicine	22.673	223,588
Nature Genetics	22.568	4500†
Pharmacological Reviews	22.524	2277
Science	22.067	165,000
Immunology Today	22.047	4000
Microbiology Reviews	20.754	11,860
Trends in Neurosciences	20.194	6000
Neuron	18.348	NA
Annual Review of Neuroscience	17.953	NA
Genes and Development	17.334	NA
Lancet	17.332	40,000*
Endocrine Reviews	17.089	4800
Trends in Pharmacological Sciences	17.013	4000
Trends in Biochemical Sciences	16.743	NA
Physiological Reviews	16.286	3300
Advances in Immunology	15.286	NA
FASEB Journal (Federation of American Societies for Experimental Biology)	15.115	24,000
Journal of Experimental Medicine	13.862	3769
Archives of General Psychiatry	11.416	38,500
Annals of Internal Medicine	9.887	95,000†
Circulation	8.634	25,000
American Journal of Human Genetics	8.598	4800
Journal of Clinical Investigation	8.467	6237
Annals of Neurology	7.624	8700
Gastroenterology	7.251	16,494
Circulation Research	6.971	3750
JAMA (Journal of the American Medical Association)	6.863	372,000
Diabetes	6.260	10,000
American Journal of Pathology	5.529	4500
Diabetologia	4.988	NA
American Journal of Psychiatry	4.570	44,000
BMJ (British Medical Journal)	4.411	112,000†
Neurology	4.347†	18,000†
Annals of Surgery	4.166	14,765
Archives of Internal Medicine	4.137	100,000
Medicine	3.900	4100

(continued)

Table 12–3. Science Citation Index* Journal Citation Reports Impact Factor for Selection of Index Medicus† Journals (1994) (*continued*)

Journal	Impact Factor†	Approximate Circulation‡
Radiology	3.800	35,684
Anesthesiology	3.660	39,168
Chemical Immunology	3.660	NA
Annual Review of Medicine	2.829	NA
Critical Care Medicine	2.807	11,000
American Journal of Medicine	2.703	53,751
Journal of Pediatrics	2.609	18,348
Archives of Surgery	2.402	39,000
American Journal of Obstetrics and Gynecology	2.247	16,491

NA = not available.

* Data provided by the journal editor or staff; figure reflects paid circulation.

† Source for impact factor information and *Index Medicus* status: *1994 Science Citation Index Journal Citation Reports*. Philadelphia (PA): Institute for Scientific Information; 1995.

‡ Source for circulation figures: *Ulrich's International Periodicals Directory*. 34th ed. New Providence (NJ): RR Bowker; 1996.

Table 12–4. Approximate Acceptance Rate for Unsolicited Manuscripts for a Selection of Medical Journals (1995)

Journal	Approximate Percentage Of Unsolicited Manuscripts Accepted	Impact Factor*	Approximate Circulation†	Index Medicus* Status
New England Journal of Medicine	7%	22.673	223,588	Yes
Journal of Bone and Joint Surgery (American Volume) (9% clinical, 4% basic)	9%‡	1.462	38,260	Yes
Lancet	9%‡	17.332	40,000	Yes
JAMA (Journal of the American Medical Association)	10%	6.863	372,000	Yes
Journal of Clinical Psychiatry	10%‡	‡3.130	32,600	Yes
Journal of Bone and Joint Surgery (British Volume)	13%‡	1.264	27,000	Yes
Annals of Internal Medicine	14%‡	9.887	95,000	Yes
BMJ (British Medical Journal)	15%‡	4.411	112,000	Yes
Pediatrics	15%‡	2.840	55,000	Yes
Academic Medicine	20%‡	1.124	5800	Yes
Nature Genetics	20%‡	22.568	3000	Yes
American Journal of Infection Control	21%‡	0.745	15,000	Yes

(continued)

Table 12–4.   Approximate Acceptance Rate for Unsolicited Manuscripts for a Selection of Medical Journals (1995) (*continued*)

Journal	Approximate Percentage Of Unsolicited Manuscripts Accepted	Impact Factor°	Approximate Circulation†	Index Medicus° Status
Journal of the American College of Cardiology	22%‡	6.013	30,500	Yes
American Family Physician	25%‡	0.354	150,000	Yes
American Journal of Ophthalmology	27%‡	1.780	17,500	Yes
Gastroenterology	28%	7.251	16,494	Yes
American Journal of Surgery	29%	1.927	15,131	Yes
American Journal of Pathology	30%‡	5.529	4500	Yes
Critical Care Nurse	30%‡	NL	95,000	No
Neurology	30%‡	4.347	18,000	Yes
American Journal of Obstetrics and Gynecology	33%‡	2.247	16,491	Yes
Journal of Rheumatology	35%‡	2.276	3400	Yes
American Journal of Clinical Pathology	40%‡	2.181	15,323	Yes
American Journal of Gastroenterology	40%‡	1.856	9620	Yes
American Journal of Nephrology	40%‡	0.961	2900	Yes
Journal of Ultrasound in Medicine	47%‡	0.807	NA	Yes
American Journal of Geriatric Psychiatry	50%‡	NL	NA	No
American Journal of Physical Medicine & Rehabilitation	50%‡	0.927	4600	Yes
Journal of Medical Microbiology	55%‡	1.627	NA	Yes
Mayo Clinic Proceedings	64%‡	1.814	95,588	Yes

NL = not listed in the *Science Citation Index*† *Journal Citation Reports*; NA = not available.

° Source for impact factor information and *Index Medicus* status: *1994 Science Citation Index* † *Journal Citation Reports*. Philadelphia (PA): Institute for Scientific Information; 1995.

† Source for circulation figures: *Ulrich's International Periodicals Directory*. 34th ed. New Providence (NJ): RR Bowker; 1996.

‡ Data provided by the journal editor or staff; figures are meant to reflect paid circulation, but some figures include unpaid circulation as well.

reference librarian at your medical library for the *Science Citation Index/Journal Citation Reports* (Garfield 1995; also see SCI/JCR in Appendix D). The printed guide to the microfiche edition ranks journals by impact factor within different medical specialties.

To find the circulation size for a journal that is not listed in Tables 12–2 through 12–5, ask your reference librarian for *Ulrich's International Periodicals Directory* (see Appendix D).

To determine whether a journal is included in *Index Medicus*, see the *List of Journals Indexed in Index Medicus* (see NIH and NLM in Appendix D). In January 1996, there were 3148 journals included in *Index Medicus*. Although many medical researchers ignore these lists, if you want your message to reach a large audience, these sources should be helpful.

Table 12–5. Prestige Factor for a Selection of Refereed *Index Medicus* Journals	
Journal	*Prestige Factor**
New England Journal of Medicine	5.069
Science	3.641
JAMA (Journal of the American Medical Association)	2.553
Annals of Internal Medicine	0.939
Nature	0.785
Lancet	0.693
Journal of Investigative Medicine	0.675
Cell	0.607
(BMJ) British Medical Journal	0.494
Archives of General Psychiatry	0.440

* The prestige factor was calculated by multiplying the circulation size by the impact factor and dividing the product by 1 million.

Many manuscripts are rejected because the editors consider the material inappropriate for their journal. However, as you probably know, submitting the same paper to more than one journal simultaneously is highly unethical. See the *New England Journal of Medicine* for a clear set of guidelines on redundant publications (Kassirer and Angell 1995) if you are in doubt about what is redundant.

GUIDELINES FOR AUTHORS

PRINCIPLE 46. READ AND FOLLOW YOUR TARGET JOURNAL'S INSTRUCTIONS FOR AUTHORS.

Follow the *Uniform Requirements for Manuscripts Submitted to Biomedical Journals* (see Appendix A) for general concepts, but more importantly, read and follow your target journal's instructions for authors. If you do not have access to the journal, editors usually are willing to send these instructions to you. When you call the editor, ask for any additional guidelines or style sheets. The alternative is to request a copy of these instructions through interlibrary loan. Many journals now provide a detailed electronic version of their guidelines for authors on the Internet (see Appendix D).

Editors and reviewers report that most authors do not adhere to the journal's format and policy. As one reviewer commented, "You must follow a rigid and unimaginative style of presentation and thinking if you wish to publish in respected (but stuffy) journals."

PLANNING THE LENGTH OF YOUR MANUSCRIPT

PRINCIPLE 47. PLAN TO SUBMIT AN ARTICLE THAT IS SHORTER THAN THE AVERAGE ARTICLE PUBLISHED IN THE TARGET JOURNAL.

See Figure 12–1, which is probably the most important graph in this book, and read several articles in the target journal, especially original research papers.

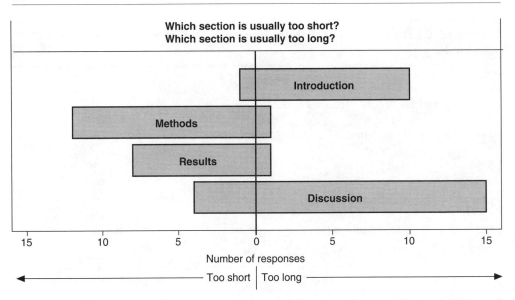

Figure 12–1. Sections of a manuscript that are too long and too short. From the Peer Review Questionnaire in Appendix B (among 29 respondents, 25 answered question 5, and 27 answered question 6).

As was mentioned in the ten key principles (see Chapter 1), the length of your manuscript should be close to the target journal's average and, ideally, slightly shorter. The number of tables, figures, and references also should be close to the average.

◎ VITAL POINT

When in doubt, make it shorter.

Use short sentences and paragraphs. The best papers are concise. When asked which section of a manuscript usually is too short, one editor answered: "None!"

Some journals measure article length by word count. The *New England Journal of Medicine* requires manuscripts to be less than 3000 words. The *British Medical Journal* limits original papers to "no longer than 2000 words, with a maximum of six tables or illustrations."

The editor of the *British Medical Journal* said that the ideal manuscript is 10 double-spaced pages, or 3 published pages, with 25 references. Some journals charge authors $150 for each excess page in the final journal format. Some journals also charge for excess figures and tables.

Authors address length limitations in two ways. Some authors write their findings, submit them for each coauthor to edit, and incorporate all of the changes into the final version, cutting material as necessary. Others set page limits for each section before they begin to write (see Table 12–1).

⊙ VITAL POINT

Estimate three to four double-spaced manuscript pages for each printed page in a journal (Table 12–6).

Plan the scope of your paper in detail. A detailed plan will help you to avoid writing a manuscript that is too long or too complex, or has too many references.

Your paper should read like a published research report, not a dissertation, so do not include too many variables. Remember, your goal is to convince the reader, as simply as possible, of the accuracy of your data and the utility of your results. As the distinguished pathologist Rudolf Virchow observed: "Brevity in writing is the best insurance for its perusal"(*Familiar Medical Quotations* 1968).

Many researchers base the first paper that they submit for publication on their thesis or dissertation. Shortening this work to an acceptable length for publication is difficult. Ask your advisor for permission to write your thesis or dissertation in two parts: an original research paper and a literature review, with all additional material placed in appendixes. This format makes it much easier to submit your thesis or dissertation for publication as two separate manuscripts. A change in medical and graduate school requirements for theses and dissertations to accommodate this two-part format (two manuscripts of publication length and quality) would have two benefits:

1. Students would learn how to write a publishable paper.
2. Students' findings would reach a broader audience.

Table 12–6. Planning Manuscript Length

Number of Double-Spaced Pages		Printed Pages	Number of Words	
Text Only°	Total†		Text Only	Total†
Short				
2–4	3–5	1	750	850
5–7	6–9	2	1500	1700
Average				
8–10	10–14	3	2250	2550
11–16	15–20	4	3000	3400
17–18	21–23	5	3750	4250
Long				
19–20	24–26	6	4500	5100
21–23	27–28	7	5250	5950
24–29	29–32	8	6000	6800
30–35	33–39	9	6750	7650
36–45	40–50	10	7500	8500

° Text only estimates include only the abstract and text (Introduction through Discussion).

† Total estimates include the title page, abstract, text, references, tables, and figures.

⊕ FOR MORE INFORMATION

The *Publication Manual of the American Psychological Association* (APA 1994) offers advice for converting a dissertation into a journal article.

WORKING WITH REVIEWERS AND EDITORS

PRINCIPLE 48. KEEP REVIEWERS HAPPY.

Table 12–7 offers suggestions for keeping reviewers happy.

Figure 12–2 ranks the reasons for outright rejection of manuscripts. The respondents said that poor methods and inadequate results were most often responsible for rejection. In contrast, Abby et al. (1994) reported that the most common reason for rejection was weak conclusions and discussion.

Table 12–7.   How to Avoid Annoying a Reviewer*

Methods

- Show a good methodology and experimental design.
- Define the research question.

Results

- Identify the key elements in the text, and consider placing them in tables.
- Use simple, easy-to-read tables and figures.
- Simplify busy tables.

Presentation

- Present the data in an unbiased manner, and let the reader come to his own conclusions before interpreting the data in the Discussion.
- Organize the paper logically.
- Follow the rules of standard English usage.
- Be concise.
- Be sure the manuscript flows.
- Prepare the manuscript carefully.
- Correct all typographical errors.
- Avoid unnecessary complexity.
- Select and display good summary information.

Statistical analysis

- Use appropriate analyses.

(continued)

Table 12–7. How to Avoid Annoying a Reviewer* (*continued*)

- Avoid, or control for, clear-cut bias.
- Explain all statistical methods clearly.
- Eliminate all statistical "snow jobs."

Discussion

- Explain the clinical relevance of the findings.

Originality

- Submit only work that has never been published.

Conclusions

- Explain how the evidence will be used.

Adherence to the journal's instructions

- Follow the journal's instructions for authors.
- Avoid having authors outnumber subjects.

° Paraphrased from answers provided to question 29 of the Peer Review Questionnaire in Appendix B.

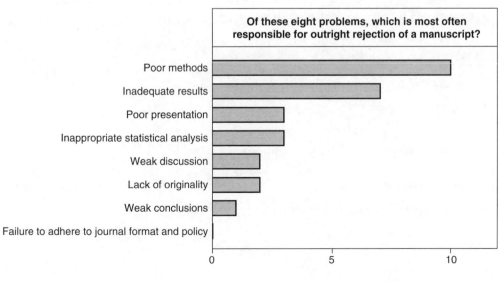

Figure 12–2. General problems responsible for rejection of manuscripts submitted for publication. From question 16 of the Peer Review Questionnaire in Appendix B.

PRINCIPLE 49. KEEP EDITORS TICKLED PINK.

Editors were bothered by many of the problems that reviewers mentioned, but editors were more concerned than reviewers about inappropriate statistical analysis. Table 12–8 gives specific suggestions for working with editors.

One editor wrote: "I get a lot of foreign manuscripts. I have learned to be patient with these authors, but I have absolutely no patience with English-speaking authors who send in poorly written manuscripts."

Table 12–8.   How to Avoid Annoying an Editor*

Methods

- Demonstrate a flawless study design.
- Clearly identify the problem, and develop it logically with the research process.

Results

- Limit the number of figures and tables.
- Describe the tables and figures adequately.
- Verify that the tables and figures agree with the text.

Presentation

- Include an accurate summary of the results, correct inferences, and appropriate discussion of both random and systematic error.
- Be clear, brief, and interesting.
- Ensure that the study is logical, with no obvious leaps.
- Organize the paper logically.
- Check spelling and grammar.
- Present the manuscript neatly and carefully.
- Eliminate redundancy.
- Use clear, precise language.
- Proofread the manuscript before submission.

Statistical analysis

- Include appropriate statistical analysis.
- Avoid technologic "pyrotechnics."
- Show that you understand your statistical analysis.

(continued)

Table 12–8. How to Avoid Annoying an Editor* (*continued*)

Discussion

- Do not repeat information in the Introduction, Discussion, and Conclusions.
- Explain the importance of the findings in a balanced way.
- Demonstrate an ability to understand the point.

Originality

- Explain the clinical relevance of the data.
- Show clinical correlation and follow-up.

Conclusions

- Be sure that the conclusions are completely supported by the Results and Methods.
- Include a well-written narrative and careful conclusions, based on a good study design.

Adherence to the journal's instructions

- Prepare the manuscript according to the journal's instructions for authors.
- Follow the journal's format for the reference section.
- Follow the correct style for the target journal.

* Paraphrased from answers provided to question 29 of the Peer Review Questionnaire in Appendix B.

As you can see from Figure 12–3, the most common problems were poor presentation and weak discussion.

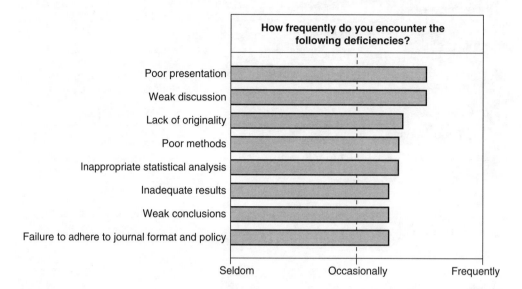

Figure 12–3. Frequency of general problems with manuscripts submitted for publication. From question 15 of the Peer Review Questionnaire in Appendix B. Because all these problems occur frequently, there is little difference among the means. However, these results can help you to focus on the most common problems.

When you have planned your study thoroughly, you are ready to move on to the second phase of the POWER principles: Observing.

P
O B S E R V I N G
W
E
R

Key Questions to Answer in the Observing Phase:

- *What if the study does not go as planned?*
- *How do I analyze these numbers?*

CHAPTER 13.

Collecting Data

MAKING OBSERVATIONS

PRINCIPLE 50. COLLECT THE DATA.

After you have stated the problem, formulated the hypothesis, and designed the study, the next step in the scientific method is to collect your data or, in other words, make your observations. In this observing phase of your project, you obtain and record your findings. For experimental studies and randomized trials, in addition to observing, you manipulate exposure or treatment. Whichever study design you choose, recognizing the common pitfalls that occur during the observing phase will prepare you for the process of writing a publishable paper.

Successful research requires periodic monitoring of the study's progress. To ensure that the study is on track, the research team should meet regularly during the observing phase, either monthly or weekly, to ensure that the protocol is being followed, the data are complete and accurate, and the members of the team agree on all major points.

KEEPING CAREFUL RECORDS

PRINCIPLE 51. RECORD YOUR RESEARCH DECISIONS AS YOU CONDUCT THE STUDY.

Writing within a well-organized framework will help readers to understand and follow the logic of your decisions. To build this framework, keep notes as you conduct the study and perform the data analysis to construct a chronological record of the project.

Create a binder of the following information:

1. The notes detailing your research decisions
2. The protocol along with any data coding conventions and abstracting guides
3. A blank data collection form
4. A full copy of each paper that you plan to use as a reference in your paper
5. The instructions for authors from the target journal
6. A recent article from the target journal

Keeping this information together and easily accessible will save you time. The statistician also will need this information during the analysis. Check with other members of your research team periodically to verify that you are all trying to answer the same research question. Record when and why your research team made major research decisions so that when you write the paper, you can describe these decisions clearly.

Be prepared to describe your decisions in sequential order, or reviewers may question your logic. For example, explain in detail why you excluded certain patients from the study. You had to solve the research problems in certain logical steps, so do not expect readers to understand the study in any other illogical sequence.

If your study involved unusual chemical substances, record their source, purity, potency, and lot number. For animal subjects, record details such as strain and supplier.

Use a word processing program to record your notes and references in a file that is structured as a manuscript (i.e., Introduction, Methods, Results, Discussion, and references). With this approach, you will avoid redundant work and your paper will be one-third finished before the analysis is completed. Remember, reviewers will be looking for a coherent framework in your study. This preparation will help them to find it.

PRINCIPLE 52. FOLLOW THE ELIGIBILITY CRITERIA PRECISELY.

During the course of the study, the research team should ensure that the planned inclusion and exclusion criteria are being followed precisely as written in the protocol. Any changes should be made democratically, and the rationale for them should be well documented. Both the statistical and clinical implications of changes in eligibility must be considered carefully. Document the number of, and reasons for, missing eligible patients.

PRINCIPLE 53. SPECIFY THE RANDOMIZATION METHODS THAT YOU USED.

To avoid ambiguity, explain in detail how randomization was conducted. For example, what was the temporal relation between randomization and treatment decisions? Describe the use of any "blocking" (randomization of subsets; for example, randomizing within each racial group or hospital).

State which subjects were "blinded," during which phase, and to what information. During some blinded studies, participants discover which group they are assigned to and therefore become "unblinded." This situation must be described honestly.

Use blinding whenever it is ethical and improves your study, especially if the outcome variable is subjective. Use double-blinding when you can, evaluate how well it worked, and report your results carefully.

DETECTING POTENTIAL PROBLEMS

PRINCIPLE 54. RECORD THE DETAILS OF INTERVENTIONS AND COMPLIANCE.

Compliance is the degree to which patients followed a physician's orders. Poor compliance among research subjects can create serious bias problems. Document and report compliance levels so that readers can draw sound conclusions. For randomized clinical trials, it is particularly important to explain how you monitored compliance with both interventions.

For studies of surgical procedures, describe the indications for the procedure and also the preoperative and postoperative conditions. Verify that you described the procedure accurately.

⊕ FOR MORE INFORMATION

See Spilker (1991).

PRINCIPLE 55. DISTINGUISH BETWEEN MISSING DATA AND THE ANSWER "NO."

A problem sometimes arises when researchers record the occurrence, but not the absence, of outcome. The data analyst does not know whether a blank means "no" or indicates a missing value. To avoid this problem, **record the absence, not just the presence, of an outcome.** For surveys, provide options for "I don't know" or "undecided" so that these responses are not confused with missing data.

PRINCIPLE 56. MONITOR THE SAMPLE SIZE.

During a study, the research team may need to reevaluate the sample size. After some information is collected, investigators often have more realistic estimates of prevalence and incidence. Recalculating the sample size in accordance with these new estimates may help your research team to project a more realistic time frame. In addition, researchers often overestimate the number of recruitable patients, so monitor the sample size while there still is money in the budget to correct problems.

CHAPTER 14

Analyzing Data: Statistical Analysis

LAYING THE GROUNDWORK FOR STATISTICAL ANALYSIS

PRINCIPLE 57. BUILD A DATABASE WITH STATISTICAL ANALYSIS IN MIND.

A common problem among medical researchers is finding an appropriate and efficient technique for data entry. Entering data in a spreadsheet is inefficient for most large clinical research projects; using database management software is usually more appropriate. Database software makes it easier to enter data and can prevent many forms of data entry errors. For small projects with fewer than 100 patients and fewer than 25 variables, you can enter data in a spreadsheet or directly into a statistical package.

Whichever software package you use, when you enter data, use exact measurements. Avoid using subjective judgments that cannot be reproduced; if you cannot avoid subjective evaluations, at least give these variables numeric codes (e.g., 0 = no, 1 = yes). Enter mutually exclusive data, such as "the most severe stage of the patient's disease" as one variable (Stage 1–4), not as separate variables (e.g., Stage 1: yes or no; Stage 2: yes or no . . .).

Sometimes, despite careful planning, you obtain text data. When you build your database, look for ways to convert these data to numbers.

Make all necessary clinical research decisions before you begin to enter data. For example, did the patient have a Grade 2 or a Grade 3 pressure ulcer? Do not enter "2–3" and then wait until the analysis is performed to classify the patient.

Entering data as text and without proper planning limits the value of your database. Remember that recoding a database is expensive. Because computer memory and speed are no longer issues, it is not necessary to record data in the least possible space. Recording data in a format that a statistical package can use for multivariate analysis (specifically, a format that will answer your research question) is more important than conserving memory.

A common mistake is to ask a programmer or medical student with no data analysis experience to develop a custom database. These people often include "bells and whistles" (unnecessary features that make the program look sophisticated), but produce a database that cannot be analyzed. It is best to have someone with years of experience in analyzing data decide how the variables will be stored and oversee database design from the beginning. For most clinical research projects, creating a database with database management software is far better than hiring a programmer to customize a database with a low-level programming language.

Label each variable in the database (or spreadsheet) program with a logical, easy-to-remember field name that will be valid for the statistical software (i.e., eight characters or fewer, no spaces, and a letter at the beginning). Using these field names simplifies the translation between the database and statistical software. After your data are completely entered into the database program, transfer the information to a statistical software package for the data analysis. Run a report in the database program or use "save as" to create a file that the statistical package can import (e.g., Lotus 1–2–3, Excel).

⊕ FOR MORE INFORMATION

If you have trouble translating files between software packages, you can use the software program DBMS/COPY by Conceptual Software and Data Junction by Tools & Techniques (see Appendix D). These software packages allow you to translate your files into someone else's format or to translate someone else's files into a software package that you prefer. The most recent version of SPSS also can import and export computer files for a variety of software packages.

Most statistical packages can read ASCII files. (ASCII is an abbreviation for the American Standard Code for Information Interchange, and is pronounced "ăs'-kē.") If you transfer your data with ASCII files, the following suggestions will simplify the process:

- Store all data in one ASCII file.
- Make each row a case (i.e., each patient or unit of analysis is entered on a separate line).
- Place each variable in a different column.
- Align decimal points vertically in columns. Data in a fixed-field format (Table 14–1) are easier to work with than data in a free-field format (Table 14–2).
- Do not use scientific notation.
- Convert measurements that are extremely small or extremely large to a scale with absolute values between 1 and 1000. For example, convert 0.0000023 gram to 2.3 micrograms.
- Assign patients to their correct groups before you enter any data. Moreover, because ambiguous values (e.g., 25%–50%) cannot be analyzed, use actual values rather than ranges or inequalities. For example, the actual age is better than < 65 versus ≥ 65. You can collapse into categories later, but you cannot "uncollapse" categories.
- For biomechanical engineering studies, calculate the average for variables that are measured repeatedly, in real time, or continuously.
- Assign codes (e.g., 99, −1) to missing values, or leave them blank.
- Code results consistently. If "no" is coded as 0 for one question, be sure that "absent" is coded as 0 for the other questions. For example:

Perinatal mortality: 0[] No 1[] Yes
Diabetes: 0[] Absent 1[] Present

- Always use a unique sequential case number to identify each patient.

Table 14–1. Example of a Fixed-Field Format File

CASE	GROUP	BPs	SEX	RACE	AGE	LOS	ICU
1	3	120	1	1	24.6	22	9
2	2	80	2	3	0.5	15	1
3	3	130	1	5	−99.9	10	0

Table 14–2.   Example of a Free-Field Format File
1,3,120,1,1,24.6,22,9   2,2,80,2,3,0.5,15,1   3,3,130,1,5,−99.9,10,0

Some medical research data files become so large that they cannot be stored on a single diskette. One solution is to compress the data files with a program known as PKZIP from PKWARE (see Appendix D); however, the person who will uncompress (PKUNZIP) the file must have the same version of the program, or a higher version.

Example 14–1.

The following command compresses the files from the directory C:\CANCER onto multiple diskettes:

C:\PKZIP\PKZIP A:\CANCER.ZIP C:\CANCER*.* -&

The following command uncompresses the files from a diskette onto the hard disk:

C:\PKZIP\PKUNZIP A:\CANCER.ZIP C:\CANCER

PREPARING THE DATA

PRINCIPLE 58. "Clean" and then "freeze" the data well in advance of your deadline.

Before you perform any analysis, use a statistical software package to perform frequencies and cross-checks to screen the data thoroughly and detect potential problems. Most databases contain many types of human and mechanical errors. **Do not skip this important step.** Although you may have deadlines and limited free time, if you hurry to analyze your data, you will be constantly repeating the analysis as you uncover one error at a time. For this reason, invest enough time and effort to clean the data completely.

Budget your time backward from your deadline. Determine how much time you need for writing, creating graphs, performing analysis, cleaning, collecting data, and planning. After data for the first 10 patients are entered, check the accuracy and completeness of the data. Meet with your research team to discuss any problems. For long-term projects, clean the data periodically by checking all inconsistencies and correcting errors.

During the planning phase, you should have identified strategies to prevent many errors, such as upper and lower limits for age in the data entry screen. However, some errors always occur, despite the most careful planning, so expect them.

Cleaning is needed when data are stored using different units (e.g., age is recorded in years, months, and weeks). Recording age in years with one decimal place usually is adequate. For example, a 6-month-old infant's age would be recorded as 0.5 (years), and a 7-month-old infant's age would be recorded as 0.6 (7/12). But you can program your database to calculate this exact age from the date of birth and the date of admission.

You can simplify the cleaning process by recording the case number on each data collection form and all related laboratory slips or monitoring strips. Filing these forms in case number order will make it much easier to check suspicious values.

Complete any missing data, or code it as "unknown." Correct the original source of the data (the database or spreadsheet), and transfer the corrected data back to the statistical package. Check with the research team to determine whether any cases should be excluded from the analysis because essential data are missing.

Document any changes made in the data and include this information in your research binder.

After the database is completely cleaned, the research team should agree to freeze the data. *Freezing the data* means that no data will be added or changed during the next phase of the analysis. Freezing the data saves time and money, but freezing uncleaned data obviously is a waste of time.

⊕ FOR MORE INFORMATION

See Chapter 15 of Hulley and Cummings (1988).

AVOIDING COMMON PROBLEMS

PRINCIPLE 59. LEARN HOW TO AVOID COMMON STATISTICAL PROBLEMS.

Someone once said: "Nature speaks but one language, and that language is mathematics." Unfortunately, many medical researchers either have avoided learning or have forgotten the language of mathematics, particularly the language of statistics. Because many health care professionals do not learn how to use statistics as part of their formal education, mastering statistics often requires self-education. Fortunately, personal computers and modern statistical software now make statistical analysis much easier and more interesting to learn.

⊕ FOR MORE INFORMATION

The SPSS software manuals (Norusis 1996) are an excellent source of information about statistical analysis. Four other books that provide a good introduction to statistics are: *Practical Statistics for Medical Research* (Altman 1991), *Basic and Clinical Biostatistics* (Dawson-Saunders and Trapp 1994), *Basic Statistics for the Health Sciences* (Kuzma 1992), and *Basic Statistical Analysis* (Sprinthall 1997).

CHAPTER 15.

Interpreting the Data

PREPARING FOR DATA ANALYSIS

PRINCIPLE 60. INTERPRET THE DATA.

After you collect and enter the data and correct the errors, you are ready to analyze the data. Interpretation is the fifth step in the scientific method. Because this analysis is still part of the observing phase, remember to keep an open mind and let the numbers reveal the truth. Do not try to force the numbers to prove your point. Analyzing the results of a clinical research study can be complicated; therefore, asking an experienced and creative data analyst for guidance almost always is prudent. Even Einstein consulted mathematicians.

The key is to find a data analyst who has adequate experience, an understanding of statistics, sufficient time, and the motivation to help you. To find such a person, ask a well-published colleague for a referral. Avoid the mistake that many medical researchers make: they do not allot sufficient time, money, or resources for data analysis. Although statistical software now is fairly easy to use, you cannot simply press a button and have the computer analyze your data. The following sections describe the more common statistical pitfalls.

PRINCIPLE 61. CREATE EQUAL-SIZED GROUPS OF PATIENTS FOR CONTINUOUS VARIABLES.

You may find that you do not have enough data or that you have an inappropriate distribution of data to perform the analysis that you originally planned. For many continuous variables, the solution to this problem is to organize your subjects into quartiles, quintiles, or deciles (4, 5, or 10 groups with approximately the same number of subjects). For example, groupings of patients by age decades (e.g., 0–9, 10–19, 20–29 . . .) might be replaced by deciles (e.g., 0–6.4, 6.5–14.9, 15.0–22.7 . . .). Quartiles, quintiles, and deciles allow you to use more effective statistical tools because they increase the likelihood of having a sufficient number of patients in each subgroup. Then, to assess the data, you can use more powerful statistical tests, such as the Mantel-Haenszel test for a linear association and the one-way analysis of variance (ANOVA).

Example 15–1.

When patients are grouped by age decades, investigators rarely have enough patients between 90 and 99 years of age to permit appropriate analysis. Yet, using deciles, the oldest 10% of patients always are grouped together. This grouping generally creates an ample subgroup. If even this group is too small, you can use quintiles or quartiles.

To decide how to regroup your data, use statistical software to create a frequency histogram.

AVOIDING COMMON PROBLEMS

PRINCIPLE 62. AVOID COMMON PROBLEMS WITH DATA ANALYSIS.

A Nobel Prize winner said that most data analysis errors occur when researchers make the following mistakes:

- They do not apply common sense to the data.
- They do not try to repeat experiments.
- They have poorly matched control groups.

PRINCIPLE 63. USE EPIDEMIOLOGIC METHODS TO MAKE THE ANALYSIS AND PRESENTATION OF YOUR DATA MORE SOPHISTICATED.

Epidemiology is the study of the spread and cause of diseases and injuries in a human population. Originally, epidemiologists studied epidemics, but now most focus on clinical research and prevention. Many epidemiologic techniques can be used to strengthen clinical research papers. Here are just three examples:

1. Person-years
2. Survival analysis and follow-up life tables
3. The dose–response relationship

Person-years are "the sum of the number of years that each member of a population has been afflicted by a certain condition (e.g., years of treatment with a certain drug)" (*Stedman's Medical Dictionary* 1995).

Because the results might be misleading in some situations, carefully consider the use of person-years if you answer "no" to any of the following questions:

- During the study period, was the risk of death or disease constant?
- Consider patients who were lost to follow-up. Was their risk of death or disease different from that in those who remained in the study?
- Did patients ordinarily survive longer than a year?

⊕ FOR MORE INFORMATION

See Mausner and Kramer (1985).

Survival analysis and follow-up life tables can be used to compare groups that are followed up for varying periods. These techniques also can be used for many other clinical problems besides survival. They allow you to adjust for varying lengths of follow-up and use the maximum amount of follow-up information, even from patients who are lost to follow-up (see principle 42). Before you collect data that require survival analysis, consult a data analyst who has experience with this technique.

For survival analysis, be sure to record:

- whether the outcome of interest occurred.
- the date of outcome.
- the date of first diagnosis.
- the date of last follow-up.
- whether the patient was lost to follow-up.

Include several variables that measure the severity of disease and any potentially confounding factors. A thorough literature search is essential to identify all variables needed to answer the research question—convincingly. Record in detail why some respondents were lost to follow-up, and analyze how the lost patients differ from the patients who remained in the study.

⊕ FOR MORE INFORMATION

See Breslow and Day (1987), Cox (1972), Kaplan and Meier (1958), and Lee (1992).

The *dose–response relationship* is a change in the amount, intensity, or duration of exposure associated with a change in the risk of a specified outcome. This gradient effect can improve a Results section that contains only borderline evidence of cause and effect by showing that outcome changes with each small change in exposure.

Example 15–2.

The incidence of lung cancer increases with the number of cigarettes smoked per day.

CHAPTER 16.

Univariate Analysis

THE MOST COMMON UNIVARIATE TESTS USED IN MEDICAL RESEARCH

PRINCIPLE 64. MASTER THE CHI-SQUARE TEST AND THE STUDENT'S *T*-TEST.

Univariate is defined as "characterized by or depending on only one random variable" (*Merriam-Webster's Collegiate Dictionary* 1993). *Univariate analysis* is a set of mathematical tools to assess the relationship between one independent variable and one dependent variable. Most medical research data can be analyzed with two univariate tests: the chi-square test and the Student's *t*-test. If you learn how to use only two tests, learn to use these two. Figure 16–1 can help you to decide which statistical test to use.

Because univariate analysis evaluates one predictor variable at a time, it cannot simultaneously adjust for other factors, such as age. Because univariate analysis is one-dimensional, it is too simplistic for many clinical research problems. Still, it is an essential first step in data analysis.

 VITAL POINT

Never bypass univariate analysis and proceed directly to multivariate analysis. Be sure that you understand the univariate results fully before you create complex multivariate models.

Bivariate is defined as "of, relating to, or involving two variables" (*Merriam-Webster's Collegiate Dictionary* 1993). Because this term often is misused, I suggest you avoid using it.

To master the chi-square and the *t*-test, you must learn the relationship between the statistic test value, degrees of freedom, and the *P* value. The following principles should make this clear.

USING THE CHI-SQUARE TEST

PRINCIPLE 65. USE THE CHI-SQUARE TEST FOR MOST CATEGORICAL VARIABLES.

Categorical variables are the simplest to analyze because they classify (e.g., smokers versus nonsmokers) rather than measure (e.g., cigarettes per day). Figures 16–2, 16–3, and 16–4 show the concepts and terms that commonly are used with a two-by-two (2 × 2) table. The chi-square test is used to determine whether the actual proportion, in two or more groups, differs significantly from the proportion expected by chance alone.

The chi-square test is appropriate for most categorical (or nominal) variables in 2 × 2 tables, when the sample size is greater than 20 and the **expected frequency** for each cell is greater than 5. Most statistical programs automatically detect when these conditions are violated.

Type of Test	Difference/ Association	Pairing	Dependent Variable — Level of Measurement	Dependent Variable — Distribution	No. of Groups	N	Appropriate Statistical Test
Question 1	Question 2	Question 3	Question 4	Question 5	Question 6	Question 7	
Univariate	Difference	Unmatched	Interval	Normal	2		Student's t-test
			Interval	Normal	≥ 2		One-way ANOVA
			Ordinal	Nonnormal	2		Mann–Whitney U test
			Ordinal	Nonnormal	> 2		Kruskal-Wallis H test
			Nominal		2	< 20	Fisher's exact test
			Nominal		≥ 2	≥ 20	Chi-square
		Matched	Interval	Normal	2		Paired t-test
			Interval	Normal	≥ 2		Correlated F ratio
			Ordinal	Nonnormal	2		Wilcoxon signed-rank test
			Ordinal	Nonnormal	> 2		Friedman ANOVA by ranks
			Nominal				McNemar's test
	Association		Interval				Pearson's r
			Ordinal				Spearman r_s
			Nominal				Mantel-Haenszel, Cramer's V°
Multivariate	Association		Interval/ordinal				Multiple linear regression
	Difference		Interval/ordinal				ANOVA
			Nominal	Not time-dependent	2		Logistic regression
			Nominal	Not time-dependent	2		Discriminant function
			Nominal	Censored	2		Cox proportional hazards

Figure 16–1. Flowchart of common inferential statistics. To use this chart, answer the following seven questions and follow the answers from left to right on the flowchart.

1. Which type of test do you need: univariate or multivariate? (Always start with a univariate test; then you can use a multivariate test to adjust for confounding factors.)

2. Do you want to test for a difference between groups or for an association between variables?

3. Were the groups matched (paired), or were they unmatched (unpaired)?

4. What is the level of measurement for the dependent (outcome) variable? Is it nominal, ordinal, or interval?

5. Is the dependent (outcome) variable normally distributed? If your histogram forms a bell-shaped curve, assume that it is normal; otherwise, assume that it is nonnormal.

6. How many groups are there for the independent (predictor) variable?

7. What is the total sample size?

Figure 16–2. Results of a screening test in a 2 × 2 table.

Results of a screening test

		Positive	Negative
Diseased	Yes	a	b
	No	c	d

Sensitivity	$\dfrac{a}{a + b} \times 100$	Percentage of subjects with the disease who have a positive test result
Specificity	$\dfrac{d}{c + d} \times 100$	Percentage of subjects without the disease who have a negative test result
Positive predictive value	$\dfrac{a}{a + c} \times 100$	Likelihood that a positive test result indicates disease
Negative predictive value	$\dfrac{d}{b + d} \times 100$	Likelihood that a negative test result indicates absence of disease
Likelihood ratio for positive results	$\dfrac{a / (a + b)}{c / (c + d)}$	Odds of a positive test result in patients with disease versus odds of a positive test result in patients without disease
Likelihood ratio for negative results	$\dfrac{b / (a + b)}{d / (c + d)}$	Odds of a negative test result in patients with disease versus odds of a negative test result in patients without disease

Figure 16–3. Predictive value measurements.

Nevertheless, you must be alert for this problem and be careful to use Fisher's exact test (Fleiss 1981) rather than the chi-square test when the sample size is small (n < 20) or the expected frequency is less than 5 for more than one-fourth of the cells.

The *Yates continuity correction* is a variation of the chi-square formula designed for small studies. This correction increases the *P* value and makes it more difficult to prove a statistically significant difference (Sprinthall 1997). The Yates correction is controversial and is probably not appropriate for most clinical research (Conover 1974). For this reason, you should use the unadjusted (Pearson) chi-square statistic in most situations (Figure 16–5). If, for some reason, you must be especially cautious not to report any borderline differences as significant, use the Yates correction.

Results of an HIV test   **Figure 16–4.** Example of a screening test.

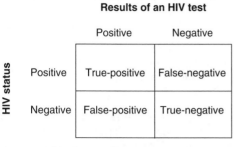

```
                       SEX
                Count
                Row  Pct   MALE       FEMALE
                Col  Pct                      Row
                            1          2      Total
      SURVIVAL
                    .00     27         36      63
      EXPIRED              42.9       57.1     6.8
                          12.3        5.0

                   1.00    192        678     870
      SURVIVED             22.1       77.9    93.2
                          87.7       95.0

                Column     219        714     933
                Total      23.5       76.5    100.0
```

Chi-Square	Value	DF	Significance
Pearson	14.13292	1	.00017
Continuity Correction	12.99934	1	.00031
Likelihood Ratio	12.44712	1	.00042
Mantel-Haenszel test for linear association	14.11777	1	.00017

```
Minimum Expected Frequency —     14.788


Number of Missing Observations:     0
```

Figure 16–5. Results of a chi-square test performed with SPSS/PC+. This figure may be confusing at first, but it provides a wealth of information, and therefore, it is worth learning how to interpret. Notice that 76.5% of the patients were female and that most of the patients who died were female, but that the mortality rate is 2.5 times higher in the male patients (12.3% versus 5.0%). The P value (listed under "Significance," on the line with "Pearson") is 0.00017. You would report this value as $P < 0.001$ and conclude that the mortality rate in male patients is higher than that in female patients and that this difference is statistically significant. Compared with women, men were 2.5 times as likely to die (relative risk 2.5, 95% CI 1.5–3.9). Also note that the P value based on the Yates continuity correction is highly significant (0.00031). See Norusis (1996) for more information.

The standard chi-square test also is inappropriate for variables with more than ordered categories (e.g., Apgar scores). For these variables, either the "Mantel-Haenszel test for a linear association" or the "Mann-Whitney U test" is more appropriate (Moses, Emerson, and Hosseini 1984). In this situation, you also can use the coefficient of contingency, or the Phi coefficient.

STATISTICAL SOFTWARE

PRINCIPLE 66. LEARN HOW TO USE A FULL-FEATURED STATISTICAL SOFTWARE PACKAGE.

The statistical software package SPSS provides a good balance of power, flexibility, and ease of use, although another statistical package may be more suited to your needs. A few of the other statistical software packages available are: BMDP, Data Muncher, Egret, Epicure, Epi Info, Genstat, GLIM, MINITAB, SAS, S-PLUS, Stata, Statgraphics, Statview, StatXact, Systat, and True Epistat (see Appendix D).

HISTOGRAMS

PRINCIPLE 67. EXAMINE THE HISTOGRAMS OF YOUR INTERVAL-LEVEL VARIABLES.

A *histogram* is a simple bar graph that shows the number of cases at each level for a particular variable. It provides you with a picture of the frequency distribution. Use your statistical package to create these histograms.

Creating a histogram for each continuous variable is the first step in analyzing interval data because it permits you to see whether your data are normally distributed, skewed, or bimodal. When you know the distribution, you can choose the correct statistical test. A normal curve has a symmetrical, bell-shaped histogram and makes it possible to use parametric tests. An asymmetrical histogram suggests that the data may be skewed and therefore require nonparametric tests. A histogram that has two peaks is called "bimodal" (see Figure 24–4). Also run frequency histograms for your categorical variables to determine whether there are variables that should be recorded.

USING THE STUDENT'S *T*-TEST

PRINCIPLE 68. LEARN HOW TO USE THE STUDENT'S *T*-TEST.

When the frequency histogram approximates a bell-shaped curve, you can use the Student's *t*-test to compare two averages, or means (Figures 16–6 and 16–7). The Student's *t*-test (also called the "independent" or "unpaired" *t*-test) can help to detect whether the means for two unmatched groups are significantly different. (If the groups are matched or the variables are measured "before" and "after" within the same patient, use the paired *t*-test.)

You can calculate the Student's *t*-test in two ways:

1. The first method assumes that the two groups have similar variances and thus pools a variance estimate for the two. (The variance is simply the standard deviation squared.)
2. The second method compares means with variances that are not similar (i.e., one group has a much larger standard deviation than the other).

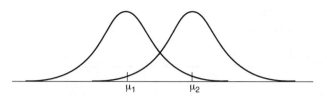

Figure 16–6. Two normal curves.

```
Independent samples of   SURVIVAL

Group 1:   SURVIVAL  EQ      .00                Group 2:   SURVIVAL  EQ     1.00


t-test for:  AGE

                      Number                      Standard      Standard
                      of Cases      Mean          Deviation      Error

         Group 1        63         85.5429         8.285         1.044
         Group 2        870        78.0354        13.631          .462
```

		Pooled Variance Estimate			Separate Variance Estimate		
F Value	2-Tail Prob.	t Value	Degrees of Freedom	2-Tail Prob.	t Value	Degrees of Freedom	2-Tail Prob.
2.71	.000	4.31	931	.000	6.58	88.44	.000

Figure 16–7. Results of a Student's *t*-test for two unpaired (unmatched) groups performed with SPSS/PC+. This test answers the question: Is the average age significantly different between the patients who died (Survival = 0, Group 1) and the patients who survived (Survival = 1, Group 2). The average age of the 63 patients who died was 85.5 years versus 78.0 years for the survivors. The standard deviations and standard errors are quite different in these two groups. Because the "2-Tail Prob." (two-tailed probability) associated with the F value is 0.000, we can assume that the variability is so large that the pooled variance estimate cannot be used. (Note that a *P* value that is less than 0.0005 is displayed as 0.000.) The separate variance estimate is used when the "2-Tail Prob." on the left is < 0.05. To describe this situation in the Results section of your paper, you might write: The patients who died were significantly older than the patients who survived (85.5 ± 8.3 years versus 78.0 ± 13.6 years, $P < 0.001$). It is also a good idea to report 95% confidence intervals. See Figure 16–8.

If *P* is less than 0.05 for the F ratio, then the variances are different enough to apply the unequal (separate) variance formula (the second method). See Figure 16–7 for an example.

With some statistical software (such as SPSS for Windows), this *P* value is displayed as "Levene's Test for Equality of Variances" (Figure 16–8). If the significance (Sig.) for this test is less than 0.05, use the results for "Equal variances not assumed." Consult your statistical software manual or see Snedecor and Cochran (1989) for more information.

Fortunately, you do not need to understand the intricacies of these statistical procedures; with most statistical software programs, running a *t*-test is easy. When two values are truly different, the difference usually is significant with both formulas.

Figures 16–8 and 16–9 demonstrate the output for a Student's *t*-test and the chi-square from SPSS for Windows (version 7.5). These correspond to Figures 16–7 and 16–5, which demonstrate the output from the DOS version of SPSS (version 4.0).

Group Statistics

	SURVIVAL	N	Mean	Std. Deviation	Std. Error Mean
AGE	EXPIRED	63	85.543	8.285	1.044
	SURVIVED	870	78.035	13.631	.462

Independent Samples Test

		Levene's Test for Equality of Variances	
		F	Sig.
AGE	Equal variances assumed	9.559	.002
	Equal variances not assumed		

Independent Samples Test

		t-test for Equality of Means						
							95% Confidence Interval of the Mean	
		t	df	Sig. (2-tailed)	Mean Difference	Std. Error Difference	Lower	Upper
AGE	Equal variances assumed	4.313	931	.000	7.507	1.741	4.091	10.923
	Equal variances not assumed	6.577	88.444	.000	7.507	1.142	5.239	9.776

Figure 16–8. Results of a Student's t-test performed with SPSS for Windows.

PRINCIPLE 69. UNDERSTAND WHEN TO AVOID USING THE STUDENT'S *T*-TEST.

When you are comparing **more than two groups,** using a Student's *t*-test repeatedly is not appropriate. Instead, use a one-way analysis of variance (ANOVA). A one-way ANOVA is used to analyze interval data and compare three or more groups. When one group has a mean that is significantly larger or smaller than that of the others, the *P* value is less than 0.05. However, to identify which groups are different, use a statistical test called the "multiple comparison procedure." Several multiple comparison procedures are available for different situations. Scheffé's procedure is a good choice for most problems.

When your frequency histogram is skewed (does not resemble a bell-shaped curve), do not use a Student's *t*-test; instead, use a nonparametric test (see Chapter 17). A typical nonparametric test will sort your data and compare the ranks instead of the actual mea-

Case Processing Summary

	Cases					
	Valid		Missing		Total	
	N	Percent	N	Percent	N	Percent
SURVIVAL *SEX	933	100.0%	0	.0%	933	100.0%

SURVIVAL * SEX Crosstabulation

			SEX		
			MALE	FEMALE	Total
SURVIVAL	EXPIRED	Count	27	36	63
		% within SURVIVAL	42.9%	57.1%	100.0%
		% within SEX	12.3%	5.0%	6.8%
	SURVIVED	Count	192	678	870
		% within SURVIVAL	22.1%	77.9%	100.0%
		% within SEX	87.7%	95.0%	93.2%
Total		Count	219	714	933
		% within SURVIVAL	23.5%	76.5%	100.0%
		% within SEX	100.0%	100.0%	100.0%

Chi-Square Tests

	Value	df	Asymp. Sig. (2-sided)	Exact Sig. (2-sided)	Exact Sig. (1-sided)
Pearson Chi-Square	14.133[b]	1	.000		
Continuity Correction[a]	12.999	1	.000		
Likelihood Ratio	12.447	1	.000		
Fisher's Exact Test				.001	.000
Linear-by-Linear Association	14.118	1	.000		
N of Valid Cases	933				

a. Computed only for a 2x2 table
b. 0 cells (.0%) have expected count less than 5. The minimum expected count is 14.79.

Figure 16–9.   Results of a chi-square test performed with SPSS for Windows.

sured values, thereby avoiding problems associated with skewed data. To compare only two groups with skewed data, use the Mann-Whitney U test. To evaluate three or more groups with skewed data, use the Kruskal-Wallis test.

To verify the results, experienced data analysts often test continuous variables with both the Student's *t*-test and the Mann-Whitney U test. Never use both these tests to fish for significance, however, because this will lead to false conclusions.

CHAPTER 17.

Nonparametric Tests

PRINCIPLE 70. KNOW WHEN TO USE A NONPARAMETRIC TEST.

Nonparametric is defined as "not involving the estimation of parameters of a statistical function" (*Merriam-Webster's Collegiate Dictionary* 1993). When data are not normally distributed or when they are on an ordinal level of measurement, nonparametric tests are appropriate. Remember, ordinal data are rankings. For example, "level of psychological stress" may be reported as: 0 = none; 1 = a little bit; 2 = moderate; 3 = quite a bit; 4 = extreme.

A common mistake in medical research is using the wrong class of statistical test, such as a parametric test in place of a nonparametric test. The basic rule is to use a parametric test for normally distributed data and a nonparametric test for skewed data. Table 17–1 lists the nonparametric equivalents for several common parametric tests.

The *Mann-Whitney U test,* the nonparametric equivalent of the unpaired Student's *t*-test, is used to compare **two groups,** but unless your data are skewed or ordinal, the Student's *t*-test is preferred and more efficient.

The rank-sum test for two independent samples ordinarily is called the "Mann-Whitney U test" (Mann and Whitney 1947). Because Wilcoxon (1945) developed an almost identical test, however, sometimes it is called the "Wilcoxon rank-sum test."

The *Kruskal-Wallis test,* the nonparametric equivalent of the one-way analysis of variance, compares ordinal or skewed data with **more than two independent groups**.

The *Wilcoxon signed-rank test,* the nonparametric equivalent of the paired *t*-test, is used only when the **two groups were matched** in some way (such as by age and sex) or when measurements were repeated within the same patient.

The *Friedman ANOVA by ranks* is the nonparametric equivalent of the correlated F ratio. This test is appropriate for assessing differences among **three or more** groups of ordinal variables that use **matching or a repeated-measures design.**

⊕ FOR MORE INFORMATION

See *Basic and Clinical Biostatistics* by Dawson-Saunders and Trapp (1994), the SPSS manuals (Norusis 1996), or *Statistical Methods* by Snedecor and Cochran (1989).

Table 17–1. Corresponding Nonparametric Tests

Parametric	*Nonparametric*
Student's *t*-test	Mann-Whitney U test
One-way ANOVA	Kruskal-Wallis H test
Paired *t*-test	Wilcoxon signed-rank test
Correlated F ratio	Friedman ANOVA by ranks

CHAPTER 18.

Matching

PRINCIPLE 71. USE MATCHING, BUT PLAN IT CAREFULLY.

Matching is an important technique for creating a control group by pairing patients based on one or more confounding factors. Matching is used when other methods of controlling for confounding variables are unsatisfactory.

Once you match patients on a variable, you cannot analyze the effect of that variable on the outcome. For this reason, be sure that you will not need to assess the effect of the matching variable. Sometimes researchers decide to match patients on age and sex without giving adequate thought to whether they need to assess the outcome effect of age and sex.

Matching is most successful and efficient when it is planned before data are collected. You can match after data are collected, but recognize the drawbacks. For one thing, time and money can be wasted collecting data on unmatched cases.

PRINCIPLE 72. DESCRIBE PRECISELY WHEN AND HOW YOU USED MATCHING.

When you report results for two comparison groups, always state whether you matched the groups in any way. Matching completely changes which statistical analyses are appropriate. As you can see from Figure 16–1, matched cases require a different set of statistical tools.

PRINCIPLE 73. CONSIDER THE HYBRID METHOD: MATCHING AND
LOGISTIC REGRESSION.

Example 18–1.

Preventable deaths are a major issue in the field of trauma care. To analyze why preventable deaths occur, investigators must control for both the severity of injury and the mechanism of injury. The typical method of mathematically weighting the effect of the severity of injury and the mechanism of injury is inappropriate because it does not adjust for the severity of injury within each mechanism group. Alternatively, patients could be analyzed in groups according to the mechanism of injury (e.g., stabbings, motorcycle crashes, falls); however, stratifying patients into these groups may make the subgroup samples so small that they are useless for statistical analysis.

One solution to this problem is the hybrid method, a statistical technique that combines matching and logistic regression to provide convincing evidence (Rothman 1986). The hybrid method is useful for statistically controlling for the severity of injury within each specific mechanism of injury. Then within the hybrid method, researchers can simultaneously consider many types of trauma patients in their analysis.

Whenever you use matching, be prepared to describe the characteristics of the unmatched group. When a bias is present, describe it and explain how it could affect the results. Some patients cannot be matched; explain why this situation is not a drawback. The final matched sample may differ significantly from the initial study group. Explain why this situation is not a bias. For instance, suppose that among fatally injured victims of motor vehicle crashes in Example 18–1, you had a person who was decapitated. Obviously, you will not find a matching survivor, but this situation does not weaken your study because the decapitated person is so severely injured that nothing can be learned about trauma care from a comparison with a survivor.

Remember, matching is an effective, but time-consuming statistical method for extracting truth from a set of numbers. In addition, it offers many advantages over using a computer program to control for confounding variables.

CHAPTER 19.

Multivariate Analysis

PRINCIPLE 74. LEARN WHEN TO USE MULTIVARIATE ANALYSIS.

Multivariate is defined as "having or involving a number of independent mathematical or statistical variables" (*Merriam-Webster's Collegiate Dictionary* 1993). "Multivariable" means the same thing, but this term is used less often and may confuse people. Unlike univariate analysis, multivariate analysis can evaluate the effect of several predictor variables simultaneously. Multivariate analysis assesses the independent contributions of multiple independent variables on a dependent variable, and identifies those independent variables most significant in explaining the variation of the dependent variable. It also permits clinical researchers to statistically adjust for differences between patients. Multivariate analysis also permits comparisons that are not mathematically independent.

Example 19–1.

Suppose that you want to determine whether the infection rate of patients who received drug A differs from that of patients who received drug B. Even though you randomized patients into two groups (A and B), you find that the patients in one group are significantly older than those in the other group. You can use multivariate analysis to adjust for the age of the patients. Then you can determine whether the infection rate differs between the two groups, independent of age.

⊕ FOR MORE INFORMATION

See Kleinbaum (1988, 1995).

PRINCIPLE 75. DESCRIBE PRECISELY HOW YOU USED MULTIVARIATE ANALYSIS TO CONTROL FOR CONFOUNDING FACTORS.

Confounding factors that are not taken into account are a common and serious statistical problem. Multivariate analysis can solve this problem by adjusting for the effects of other variables. However, to allow the reader to judge the validity of your study, you must describe—in plain English—how you controlled for confounding variables. Reviewers expect you to search the literature and study the appropriate papers. Be aware of which variables cited in the current literature are potentially confounding factors for your study. Even if you did not include these factors in your multivariate analysis, note in your paper that you are aware of them.

PRINCIPLE 76. BECOME FAMILIAR WITH LOGISTIC REGRESSION ANALYSIS.

Logistic regression is a multivariate statistical technique that is commonly applied (and misapplied) in medical research. When outcome is recorded in two categories, such as dead versus alive, logistic regression is an effective way to examine the independent contributions of more than one predictor variable. Logistic regression probably will be even more important in the future. For this reason, it is a good idea to learn how to use it or at least how to interpret it.

Hosmer and Lemeshow (1989) explained the fine points of logistic regression. If you reference their book, you can avoid describing every detail of your logistic regression analysis in your Methods. Kleinbaum (1995) also wrote a self-learning text on logistic regression. Some logistic regression techniques are too complex and lengthy to include in a medical journal article. For example, you may miss important predictor variables if you choose the typical P value threshold of less than 0.05 for variable entry. For many logistic regression models, using a less stringent P value (e.g., $P < 0.15$ or $P < 0.20$) is more appropriate for selecting variables to enter into the model.

Many researchers ignore the most valuable information provided by logistic regression: the outliers. After the predictor variables are mathematically weighted, logistic regression attempts to predict the outcome based on your model. Patients who clearly do not fit the model (outliers) are noted (e.g., infants who had a poor outcome, but were predicted to have a good outcome).

◎ VITAL POINT

Review the outliers, pull the patient charts, and interview the patients or families to learn about other factors that are not included in your model.

Example 19–2.

Examination of the outliers in one logistic regression model showed that among mothers who smoked cigarettes during their pregnancy, the infant outcome could not be predicted by the risk factors under study.

Remember, the experiment that came out wrong is trying to tell you something.

Discriminant function analysis is an older and less robust multivariate test similar to logistic regression. Discriminant function analysis sometimes causes problems with categorical independent variables. If you choose discriminant function over logistic regression, explain why.

PRINCIPLE 77. GET A SECOND OPINION BEFORE CONCLUDING THAT THERE WERE NO DIFFERENCES BETWEEN THE STUDY GROUPS.

In clinical studies, the significant findings are usually found deep in the numbers, so deep that multivariate analysis often is required to control for differences among patients. Even randomized studies based entirely on univariate analysis should not be interpreted as showing that no significant differences existed.

These problems of concluding that no differences exist commonly occur when data are analyzed by people who do not have a solid understanding of both the research subject and the statistical methods. Incorrect conclusions also can be drawn when the analysis does not examine important subgroups or does not use the proper multivariate method.

An *interaction* is the combined influence that two or more variables can have on outcome. Never overlook the importance of interactions.

Example 19–3.

A group of investigators found that among people with spinal cord injury, both diabetes and smoking were moderate risk factors for pressure ulcers. However, all of the patients who had diabetes and also smoked had a history of pressure ulcers. This effect from a combination of factors is an interaction.

PRINCIPLE 78. CLEARLY DESCRIBE THE METHODS YOU USED TO PERFORM MULTIVARIATE ANALYSIS.

Although you may use complex multivariate analysis to control for confounding factors, always simplify the presentation of the findings to make them useful for readers. Explain these results clearly, and graph the main points. This task is not easy and may be time-consuming. However, if you skip this step, reviewers may misinterpret the independent contributions of your key variables.

 VITAL POINT

Always translate multivariate analysis into plain English.

Most reviewers and editors are not statistical experts, and what they do not understand may hurt you. Their misunderstanding can lead to a rejection of your paper. To ensure that reviewers and editors understand your statistical analysis:

- Explain how you used multivariate analysis to adjust for the overlap in variables and solve the problem of confounding factors.
- Describe how you chose the variables that you used in the multivariate analysis, and explain why you did not include other variables previously associated with your measure of outcome.
- Indicate how and why you chose certain interactions and whether you examined other interactions.

PRINCIPLE 79. PRESENT THE RESULTS OF THE MULTIVARIATE ANALYSIS IN A CLINICALLY USEFUL FORMAT.

Tables of multivariate analysis should provide a balance of clinical and statistical information. These tables are most useful when they are designed jointly by clinical and statistical experts. Tables are discussed in further detail in Chapter 24.

Do not allow multivariate analysis to overcomplicate your paper. Provide a balance of multivariate results to show that you did not subjectively synthesize unseen results. **Present evidence from each major step of the analysis.** Otherwise, reviewers may suspect that you created a model that you believed was true and simply used statistics to support your opinion. A paper that does not provide this evidence demands an **unacceptable leap of faith from the reader,** and much of the science is lost by this apparent subjectivity.

 VITAL POINT

When you use several multivariate models to choose variables for a scale or an index, clearly describe how you chose the factors for the final model.

The variable selection rules should be objective, clear, quantifiable, and reproducible. Use a conceptual (rather than an empirical) basis for selecting variables into the models. For example, do not select variables based solely on *P* values; consider what makes sense clinically.

Group the potential variables into logical, clinically meaningful clusters, such as preexisting diseases, injury severity factors, time factors, and treatment factors. Then you can design multivariate models to test groups of variables in stages or blocks, according to a logical ordering system and a hierarchical design. These results will have more practical value than robotically analyzed data.

PRINCIPLE 80. LEARN COX PROPORTIONAL-HAZARDS REGRESSION.

To publish a paper in a high-quality journal, you may have to show that you adjusted for several confounding factors and for varying lengths of follow-up. The tool that you will need is Cox proportional-hazards regression. Although many researchers find it easier to subcontract this analysis, there are several reasons why you should learn how to use this technique. First, you will be able to communicate more effectively if you know the basics of building a statistical model. Second, multivariate modeling often requires a clinical judgment based on years of experience to select the optimal variables for analysis. Third, with modern statistical software, this type of analysis is actually enjoyable.

⊕ FOR MORE INFORMATION

See Cox (1972) and the SPSS Advanced Statistics manual (Norusis 1996).

PRINCIPLE 81. BECOME FAMILIAR WITH THE STATISTICAL TOOLS OF THE FUTURE.

Reviewers and editors predict that the statistical techniques shown in Table 19–1 will be increasingly important in the future.

Table 19–1.   Statistical Tools of the Future
I.   Multivariate Analysis   • Used for large samples   • Use of special bias-avoiding techniques to analyze large databases   • Analysis of variance (ANOVA)
II. Meta-analysis   Many experts said that meta-analysis would be a more important statistical tool in the future, and several mentioned the importance of learning how to use it properly, but one reviewer said that meta-analysis was inherently and fatally biased.
III. Logistic Regression
IV. Other Statistical Tools   • Cox proportional-hazards regression
(continued)

Table 19–1. Statistical Tools of the Future (*continued*)

- Generalized estimating equation (GEE; Lipsitz et al. 1994; Leger and Liang 1986)
- Exact tests
- Path analysis: multidimensional scaling
- Jackknife techniques
- Techniques to compare relative risk
- Recursive partitioning

V. Reported by Altman and Goodman (1994)

- Bootstrap
- Gibbs sampling
- Generalized additive models
- Classification and regression trees
- Models for longitudinal data
- Models for hierarchical data
- Neural networks

PRINCIPLE 82. DRAW YOUR CONCLUSIONS USING CLINICAL COMMON SENSE TO INTERPRET YOUR RESULTS.

After you analyze your results, meet with your research team and then carefully draw your conclusions. Drawing conclusions is the sixth and final step in the scientific method. When you and your research team have completed the Observing phase, you can move on to the third phase of the POWER principles: Writing.

P
O
W
E
R

WRITING

Key Questions to Answer in the Writing Phase:

- *Why did you perform the study? (Introduction)*

- *What is the research question? (Introduction)*

- *What did you do? (Methods)*

- *What did you find? (Results)*

- *What do your results mean? (Discussion)*

CHAPTER 20.

Title

PRINCIPLE 83. GIVE YOUR ARTICLE A SNAPPY TITLE.

With the planning and observing phases of your research completed, you should have most of the material you need to write your paper. Few medical manuscripts are in fact written in order, from beginning to end. However, for ease of use, the following chapters on writing your paper are organized into the sections of a typical manuscript.

The first words that a potential reader will see are those in your title, so make the title interesting and easy to understand. Table 20–1 shows the ingredients for a good title.

If your findings are not broadly applicable, be sure that the title does not suggest that they are. Compare the characteristics of your sample (e.g., age, race, sex) with those of the general population. For example, does the title explain how your sample differs from the general population? As one expert suggested: "See if your title can show how the study may enhance (or at least apply to) patient care, either now or in the future."

PRINCIPLE 84. PROVIDE THE SPECIES OF ANY ANIMAL SUBJECTS USED IN YOUR STUDY.

For studies that involved nonhuman subjects, include the species of animal or organism in the title. This level of detail allows researchers who scan the literature to decide whether the study interests them without having to retrieve the full paper.

PRINCIPLE 85. DELETE UNNECESSARY WORDS AND PHRASES FROM YOUR TITLE.

Table 20–2 shows words and phrases that often can be deleted from a title.

Table 20–1.   Elements of a Good Title
Easy to understand
Accurate promise of the paper's content
Specific concerning the scope of the study
Does not use unexplained abbreviations unless they are widely understood by the target journal's audience (e.g., HIV, AIDS, CD4$^+$, DNA, RNA, IQ)
Simple, short, concise
10 to 12 words long
Interesting
States the subject of the article, but not the conclusions
Nondeclarative
Indicates the study design
Eye-catching, a "reader-grabber" (Baker 1986)
Begins with a key word
Grammatically correct
Worded appropriately for the target journal audience

Table 20–2.   Phrases to Avoid in the Title
For all studies:

For all studies:
- A Study of
- A Study to Determine the
- An Innovative Method
- An Investigation Into
- Contributions to
- Correlations of
- Investigations on
- Means of
- Notes on
- Observations on
- Preliminary Studies of
- Report of a Case of
- Results of
- Retrospective
- Studies on
- Use of

For cross-sectional studies:
- A Test to Predict
- Cause of
- Development of
- Predictors of

CHAPTER 21.

Abstract

WRITING THE ABSTRACT

PRINCIPLE 86. TAKE THE TIME TO POLISH THE ABSTRACT.

Make a good first impression with a well-written abstract. Most people will read only your abstract, so invest plenty of time in writing it. Your abstract should demonstrate that your findings are clinically (or biologically) important and that your study was performed carefully. If necessary, ask your colleagues for feedback to identify sentences that need to be refined.

Editors will read your abstract to learn whether it is well written and whether the topic is appropriate for their journal. A good abstract is specific, representative of the article, and structured correctly for the target journal. For example, if the target journal uses a single-paragraph format, obviously, you should also.

Clearly describe the problem in the first sentence of the abstract. Describe your objective sufficiently, yet simply, and be sure that it is not too broad for a single study to answer. To help the reader understand what you are testing, include the primary null hypothesis in the abstract. Then explain how you conducted the study, and finally, describe any notable results and your primary conclusion.

Avoid using the same sentences in both the abstract and the body of the paper. Because a lack of organization often is a problem, many unstructured abstracts can be improved by using the *New England Journal of Medicine* four-section structure: Background, Methods, Results, and Conclusions.

Some researchers write the final draft of the abstract after the manuscript is completed. Others write the abstract first and use it as a guide for writing the rest of the paper. With either method, remember that preparing a good abstract always requires **extensive rewriting.**

EDITING AND REVISING THE ABSTRACT

PRINCIPLE 87. KEEP THE ABSTRACT SHORT.

Do not wait for the editor to tell you:

 The abstract is much too long.

Most journals have a section that describes the correct format for papers submitted for publication (usually called the "information for authors"). Follow these instructions exactly, and compare your format with that of abstracts published in recent issues of the target journal. Usually, structured abstracts (i.e., where a format is specified) are less than

250 words long and unstructured abstracts are less than 150 words long. Some journals (e.g., psychology journals) recommend limiting abstracts to 120 words.

Do not shorten the abstract by excluding key information. The abstract must summarize your study design and **briefly state your findings** (e.g., N = ?; the percentage with poor outcome = ?). Do not merely promise that the findings will be described in the full paper. The abstract also should briefly describe the clinical relevance of the findings.

Eliminate all abbreviations and unnecessary words. Do not use abbreviations unless you are certain that the readers of the target journal will understand them. Never cite figures or tables in the abstract. Include key words only if the target journal's instructions request them. During your literature search, you can identify appropriate key words among the MeSH (Medical Subject Headings) terms. Place these key words at the end of the abstract.

◎ VITAL POINT

Keep your conclusions specific and conservative.

CHAPTER 22.

Introduction

CAPTURING THE READER'S ATTENTION

PRINCIPLE 88. BEGIN WITH THUNDER.

Write a strong introductory paragraph, and go right to the essence of the argument to "hook" the reader. The opening sentences of the Introduction and of each section must be original "reader-grabbers" (Baker 1986). A provocative question, a new perspective, and sometimes a good quotation are useful bait for catching readers.

Sometimes all you need to do is move a word to improve the cadence, but more often, revising the Introduction takes both time and creative energy. **Be imaginative, not imitative.** A concise account of the extent, prevalence, or cost of the problem can be effective—if it is well written and interesting.

James Thurber's editor once told him to begin his newspaper articles with a short lead (Gilmore 1989). The next day, Thurber's article began:

> *"Dead. That was what the man was . . ."*

Obviously, this example is a little extreme, but you do need to consider the reviewers' point of view. They may be tired, overworked, and utterly bored with your topic. To interest them, explain why your study is necessary, and convey your enthusiasm for the work. Do not exaggerate, however, and never let your tone become emotional or hostile.

PROVIDING ADEQUATE BACKGROUND INFORMATION

PRINCIPLE 89. REFERENCE AND DEFINE BACKGROUND INFORMATION.

Start the Introduction with a general, yet concise, description of the problem that your paper will address. In the next few sentences, reference previous work that supports your assessment of the problem.

Early in the Introduction, define the primary subject of your paper. **Define any new, unusual, or vague terms used in the title or introduction, such as "poor nutritional status" or "preventable death."** If other authors have defined these terms differently, help the reader understand the differences between the definitions, and explain why you defined the terms as you did. Anticipate and avoid the following types of criticism:

 The phrase "high risk" must be applied carefully, defined, and referenced. Otherwise, the reader may wonder: "High risk for what?" "Are all patients at equally high risk?"

 Please clarify what is meant by "severe X."

How do we define this condition?

 Presumably, there is some gold standard against which we measure care. But what is it, and how is it derived?

 "Uneventful" should be defined.

◎ VITAL POINT

Define all potentially questionable terms.

You may think that definitions are not necessary because your colleagues will understand the terminology. However, today, many reviewers are statisticians and others outside your subspecialty who may not understand your terminology. Defining unfamiliar terms makes your study easier for them to understand and should improve the ratings of your paper.

PRINCIPLE 90. WRITE A CONCISE, FOCUSED INTRODUCTION.

Reviewers often complain that the Introduction is **too long** and contains too much history, too many references, and not enough punch. Avoid writing a verbose Introduction that will make reviewers moan: "Who cares?"

You can improve your Introduction by explaining why your research question is important, interesting, or controversial, but do not include paragraphs of information that can be found in a textbook. Although you may have conducted an exhaustive review of the literature, include only the most relevant and significant points in your Introduction. Anticipate criticism such as the following:

 What sensitivities, specificities, and predictive values have been reported in similar patients?

 The Introduction needs to reference the literature to show that the reported results are better than a placebo; otherwise, a reader may think: "Maybe neither drug is effective."

 What is the overall success rate for this treatment in patients with this condition?

 What is the difference between the complication rates for these groups?

What is the evidence that one factor is as important as another in causing the complication?

PRINCIPLE 91. USE THE LITERATURE TO ENRICH YOUR INTRODUCTION.

Do not over-reference the Introduction. This section in particular must be short. On the other hand, if your sample is small or if you do not have an ideal control group, you can strengthen your paper with a few well-selected findings from published studies.

In a 1995 Forbes article, the journalist Philip Ross wrote: "Flip-flops in the history of health advice are the rule rather than the exception." To avoid this type of criticism, **prove that you understand the historical importance of your subject.** Within this body of knowledge, position your study. For example, does your study have a larger sample size, better control of confounding factors, longer follow-up, more recent data, or more accurate measurements? Summarize this account as concisely as possible in the Introduction and elaborate on it in the Discussion.

◎ VITAL POINT

Point out the gap in current scientific knowledge and explain how your study fills this gap.

PRINCIPLE 92. ARTICULATE THE PURPOSE OF YOUR STUDY CLEARLY.

The study should not appear to be organized around analysis of a variety of measurements in hope of finding any significant differences. In the Introduction, provide a clear map showing the direction of your study so the reviewer does not interpret it as a "fishing trip."

Identify the major point of your paper and write to that point; do not go off on tangents. Deliver what you promise without making the reader hunt for it. **The specific aim and hypothesis should be easy to find and understand.** State when, in your research project, you developed this hypothesis.

Be sure that the reasoning in your paper follows a straight line from the purpose (in the Introduction) to the conclusion (at the end of the Discussion). Straying from the hypothesis or the objective of the analysis is a problem with many research papers. A good paper has one main problem to solve, not two or three. At the end of the Introduction, be sure to describe the overall purpose of your study, but not your conclusions.

If you have trouble deciding where to start, take four index cards, one for each major section of your paper: Introduction, Methods, Results, and Discussion. On each card, answer the question: What is the most important point of this section? Identifying these four points can help you to write a focused paper that readers will understand. If this method does not help, remember what Steve Martin said: "Writer's block is a fancy term made up by whiners so they can have an excuse to drink alcohol."

⊕ FOR MORE INFORMATION

See the *Publication Manual of the American Psychological Association* (APA 1994) for examples and further details on what is appropriate for the Introduction.

PRINCIPLE 93. CONDENSE THE INTRODUCTION.

Writing a good Introduction is a challenge because you must present a great deal of important information in just a few words. How few? Check recently published Introductions in the target journal, and make yours slightly less than or equal to the average length.

◎ VITAL POINT

Nearly all reviewers and editors agreed on the following piece of advice (see Figure 12–1): Make the Introduction shorter.

CHAPTER 23.

Methods

PURPOSE OF THE METHODS SECTION

PRINCIPLE 94. PROVIDE AMPLE DETAILS IN YOUR METHODS SECTION.

The Methods is the simplest section to write because it simply recounts what you have done. Ironically, however, the leading cause of manuscript rejection is a poor Methods section (Figures 23–1 and 23–2).

◎ VITAL POINT

Replicability of results is the heart of science, so budget sufficient time to write a complete and accurate Methods section.

The goal in writing the Methods section is to present a clear, but detailed exposition of the research design. An exceptional Methods section is an indispensable part of a successful paper. If your Methods section is less than two double-spaced pages, you probably need to add more details before you submit your paper. Reviewers often reject papers that have less than two pages of Methods.

PRINCIPLE 95. ORGANIZE THE METHODS ACCORDING TO MEANINGFUL SUBHEADINGS.

Table 23–1 shows an example of Methods subheadings. Using subheadings makes it much easier for you to write the paper and for reviewers and readers to understand it. Be sure that you use subheadings that are logical and meaningful, and that you have enough text to justify each subheading. A subheading followed by only one or two sentences of text looks peculiar.

THE STUDY DESIGN

PRINCIPLE 96. AVOID THE TERM "RETROSPECTIVE."

The Methods section should of course describe the study design and explain how the data were collected. Yet, as Kassirer and Campion (1994) pointed out, many papers are rejected because the authors did not adequately explain the experimental design. This problem also is evident in Figures 23–3 and 23–4.

Part of the problem is simply miscommunication. "Retrospective" is a word that causes much confusion. As described in Chapter 3, the term "retrospective" refers to the act or process of surveying the past, and often is based on memory. In a retrospective study, people with and without a specified outcome are compared. Researchers investigate the histories of these two groups to look for the presence of, or exposure to, a particular factor. Then the proportions of subjects with this factor are compared between the two groups.

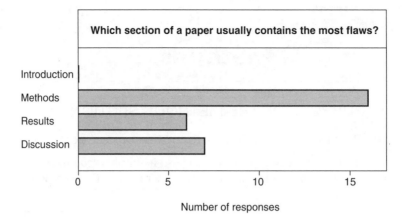

Figure 23–1. The manuscript section that usually contains the most flaws. From question 3 of the Peer Review Questionnaire in Appendix B.

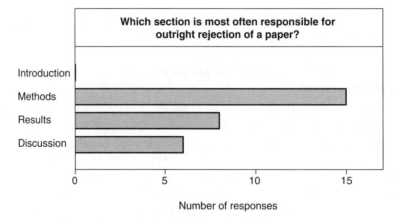

Figure 23–2. The manuscript section that is most often responsible for rejection. From question 4 of the Peer Review Questionnaire in Appendix B.

Table 23–1.   An Example of Subheadings Used in a Methods Section

Study Design
Eligibility
Randomization and Blinding
Intervention and Compliance
Assessment of End Points
Statistical Analysis

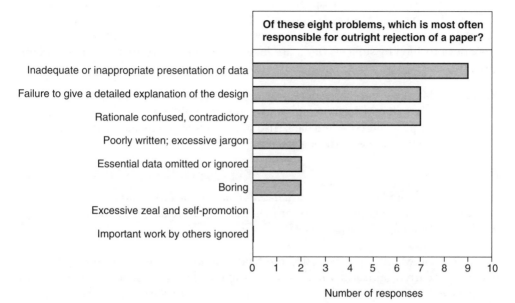

Figure 23–3. Presentation problems and rejection. From question 13 of the Peer Review Question-naire in Appendix B.

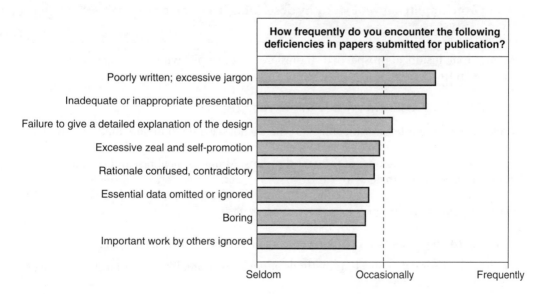

Figure 23–4. The frequency of presentation problems. From question 12 of the Peer Review Questionnaire in Appendix B.

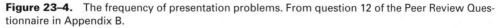

If you collected your data by surveying the past (retrospectively), explain why this approach was appropriate, despite its limitations. Retrospectively collected information often is of poorer quality than prospectively collected information because the presence or absence of many conditions is not documented consistently in routine medical records. For instance, smoking and drinking histories may be vague or may not be recorded at all. Histories provided by subjects often are inaccurate and biased. In addition, the control group may be a major limitation because it is the potential source of many types of bias.

In both the Methods and Discussion, provide information to help the editor and reviewers see why they should recommend your paper for publication rather than wait for a study with prospectively collected data. Also state whether you included observations that were recorded before the study began.

Example 23–1.

If you reported blood pressures, state whether you obtained the readings from records of previous admissions and office visits, or if all readings were observed and recorded after you began the study.

Always explain whether you recorded the study variables before or after the disease or outcome occurred and also whether you assigned the patients to the study groups prospectively or retrospectively. Also state whether you reviewed charts before or after the patients were discharged.

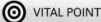 VITAL POINT

Avoid oversimplifying your study by describing it as "retrospective" or "prospective."

Many strong historical prospective studies are handicapped when investigators mislabel them as "retrospective."

PRINCIPLE 97. USE THE TERM "PROSPECTIVE" CAREFULLY.

Prospective designs begin with subjects who do not have the outcome under study. The presence of suspected etiologic factors is determined, and the subjects are followed up to see in whom the outcome of interest develops. Many medical researchers misuse the word "prospective." Instead of "retrospective" and "prospective," use more specific terms, such as "case–control," "cohort," "cross-sectional," or "historical prospective," to describe your study design.

PRINCIPLE 98. DESCRIBE YOUR DATA COLLECTION METHODS IN DETAIL.

To describe your data collection methods adequately, think like a journalist and answer the following questions:

- Who?
- What?
- When?
- Where?
- How?
- Why?

Further, describe the protocol for finding data. Without explicit details, reviewers will ask such questions as:

 Were data complete for all patients?

 How much time elapsed between hospital discharge and abstraction of the records?

Describe how you handled the problem of missing data. Extensive missing data and other quality problems will damage your manuscript's rating. Also state whether all or part of your cohort of patients was included in previous publications.

PRINCIPLE 99. SPECIFY WHO COLLECTED THE DATA.

State how many people collected the data, and describe their qualifications. Document the intra-rater and inter-rater reliability testing. Describe the steps that were taken to ensure the accuracy of the data and coding, or reviewers may ask:

 Who read the ultrasounds?

 Were the findings verified?

 Were readers "blinded" to the patients' clinical courses?

 How many persons collected the information for this study? Were conditions that developed before the implementation of the study included?

 Were these conditions documented by history from the patient or by observation?

 How accurate is the coding for preexisting conditions?

Reporting that "there was no documented history of X" usually is more accurate than claiming that a subgroup of patients "never had X."

PRINCIPLE 100. DESCRIBE THE SETTING OF THE STUDY.

Explain where the study was conducted, and provide relevant information about the institution, such as:

- What type of population is served by the hospital or institution?
- Is the setting urban, suburban, or rural?

- How many beds does the hospital have?
- Is the facility a teaching hospital?
- Is it a tertiary care center?

PRINCIPLE 101. DEFINE YOUR VARIABLES.

Carefully define important variables, grades of conditions, and criteria for disease severity. Reviewers expect that any potentially confusing terms in the title, abstract, or Introduction will be clearly defined in the Methods. Double check that you have defined all nebulous terms.

Example 23–2.

Congenital anomalies can be defined with International Classification of Diseases (ICD) codes 740.0 through 759.9. Note how this coding provides a concise, yet unambiguous definition.

The Methods must provide enough detail to enable one of your peers to reproduce your study. To ensure that it does, look for the following types of problems:

 The diagnoses are not sufficiently rigorous for us.

 How and when were measurements and determinations for the key variables made?

 How were the conditions diagnosed or classified?

 Would most experts in this field agree with these definitions?

 What protocol was followed for treatment?

 Were all three variables needed for a positive finding, or any one of the three?

 A brief description of how mobility and activity were measured is needed.

State the cutoff points for diagnosis of medical conditions. You can avoid lengthy descriptions by referencing laboratory, statistical, and scaling methods to standard works. For the reader's benefit, consider using textbooks or literature reviews rather than highly technical original papers, and include page numbers. If you modify a published method, provide enough detail to make your variation reproducible. **Finally, reference any previous publication that described your study's database, protocol, or design.**

Anticipate reviewers asking: "How much?," "How long?," and "When?" For example:

Give an indication of when the blood was drawn, and whether or not the patients were fasting at the time of blood drawing.

 The Methods need to be expanded. Tests were performed twice a week, but it is unclear which tests were included in the final analysis.

 In the Materials and Methods section, the authors describe their use of X. The authors need to be much more precise in describing how X was evaluated. If an abnormal value was detected, did the authors verify it by additional readings? Did the authors take six readings and average them? And so on.

Reviewers expect details:

 How many milligrams of the drug were injected?

 How about the size of the needle?

ELIGIBILITY

PRINCIPLE 102. DESCRIBE THE SOURCE OF THE STUDY SUBJECTS.

In the Methods, present objective inclusion criteria. State the number of patients who met your inclusion criteria. Saying, "I deemed 79 patients inappropriate," is both archaic and unreproducible, and gives the impression that you selected cases that agreed with your opinion. Keep track of which patients were excluded from the study.

State how many patients were excluded, and for what reasons. Also explain how many patients were excluded for more than one reason. If you established any priority for the exclusion criteria, explain your decision. Compare the excluded patients with the study group. In the Discussion, explain how any differences between the groups could alter the interpretation of the findings.

Anticipate the following types of concerns from reviewers:

 The authors should provide the denominator: total deliveries during the study period at the authors' institution. They also should provide the percentage of deliveries that met the inclusion criteria and the number of patients excluded.

 Were all patients delivered during the 5-year period at the institution included, and if not, how were patients selected?

⊙ VITAL POINT

Do not include results in the Methods section.

PRINCIPLE 103. PROVIDE THE BEGINNING AND ENDING DATES OF THE STUDY.

Give the dates that were used in your inclusion criteria, and explain why you chose these limits. If you later uncover a few more "good" cases that occurred outside these limits, resist the temptation to add them. Remember, your article may be read in many countries, and you can avoid confusion by spelling out the month. For example, 1/12/97 may be read as January 12, 1997, or December 1, 1997.

RANDOMIZATION AND "BLINDING"

PRINCIPLE 104. EXPLAIN YOUR RATIONALE FOR RANDOMIZING.

In the Methods section, state whether the subjects were randomly assigned to receive the treatment, and provide reproducible details of the randomization methods that you used.

Reviewers usually prefer blinded randomization. Yet, according to Fried (1974), ". . . the claims for the RCT [randomized controlled trial] have been greatly, indeed preposterously overstated." Despite reviewers' preference for randomization, randomized studies can have problems.

Example 23–3.

Suppose, for instance, that as part of a study of educational methods, class sizes were randomly set as large or small. A number of factors might affect the outcome. Teachers might change their teaching methods based on the size of the class. Consequently, the results might be caused not by the number of students in the classroom, but by the teaching method.

Reviewers may regard nonrandomized studies as too weak for publication unless you prove that the groups were similar or that you controlled for the differences between the groups.

For many clinical problems, an observational study is the only ethical alternative. These studies often are less expensive, more realistic, and more efficient than experimental studies because they answer the research question quickly. You must build your case, as a lawyer would, for observational studies.

In observational studies, the variables (e.g., class size) are not manipulated; they simply are observed in their natural state, with various conditions and various outcomes. Statisticians often prefer comprehensive observational databases to randomized controlled trials, especially to evaluate potentially lifesaving therapies (Berry 1989; Royall 1991). As Truog (1992) pointed out, for some clinical research problems, observational studies provide the optimal balance of high-quality treatment and scientific research. The "takeaway" message is to always explain your reasons for selecting your study design.

PRINCIPLE 105. DESCRIBE THE INFORMED CONSENT PROCESS USED IN YOUR STUDY.

For all randomized studies, experimental investigations, and studies that used interviews with human subjects, state whether you obtained informed consent. If you did not obtain informed consent, explain why. Demonstrate that you protected the patients' rights. If consent was not required, explain why. Many journals do not even consider manuscripts that do not address the issue of informed consent.

⊕ FOR MORE INFORMATION

See Hulley and Cummings (1988) for a discussion of informed consent and exemptions.

INTERVENTION AND COMPLIANCE

PRINCIPLE 106. PROVIDE SPECIFICS FOR ANY DRUGS OR DEVICES THAT WERE TESTED.

For studies of biomedical devices, enclose unfamiliar engineering terms in quotation marks, and define these terms specifically for the readers of the target journal. Capitalize any proprietary names (e.g., trademarks). Describe other competing medical devices, and explain why you studied that particular brand and model.

Some journals list the name of the device with the manufacturer's name, city, state, and country in parentheses. The key point to remember is that reviewers and editors will be especially concerned with potential bias and disguised advertising.

For pharmaceutical studies, provide the dosage and route of administration. As always, follow the policy of the target journal for providing drug names. Most journals use the drug's generic, or nonproprietary, name (e.g., aspirin, digitalis) in text. The first time you name each drug, include the proprietary, or trade, name (capitalized) and the manufacturer's name and location in parentheses.

PRINCIPLE 107. OMIT UNNECESSARY DETAILS.

Although computer hardware and software specifications may be an important part of your work, avoid providing superfluous details in the Methods section. In most cases, you can simply state whether you used a mainframe or a personal computer, and give the name and version of the statistical software.

PRINCIPLE 108. PROVIDE A FULL EVALUATION OF THE SCREENING TESTS.

When you compare several clinical tests, state whether the tests were diagnostic, screening, or prognostic according to the following criteria:

- *Diagnostic tests* determine the presence of a disease.
- *Screening tests* are relatively inexpensive diagnostic tests that detect individuals who need more testing.
- *Prognostic tests* predict the outcome of a disease.

If some of your patients underwent more than one test, explain the order of testing and the rationale for this order. If some of the tests were repeated, explain which results were included in the analysis and graphs. Also, explain your institution's testing protocol.

For some conditions, sensitivity is important; for others, specificity is more important. Discuss the relative importance of sensitivity and specificity for patients with the study condition. Finally, describe how many patients with an adverse outcome had more than one abnormal test result.

⊕ FOR MORE INFORMATION

See Dawson-Saunders and Trapp (1994); Fletcher, Fletcher, and Wagner (1996); and Sackett et al. (1991).

END POINTS AND OUTCOME

PRINCIPLE 109. DEFINE OUTCOME.

End points are the variables that represent the completion of a study interval (e.g., discharge from the hospital or death). The Methods section must include a reproducible, detailed description of your end points.

When using a variable as a measure of outcome, clearly define your criteria. Even if they seem obvious, define all measures of outcome. If you use a definition that differs from that found in the dictionary, provide your definition. Defining your outcome will improve the odds of publication by avoiding criticism such as the following:

My major concern continues to be the end point that you used for discharge, the patient's ability to walk independently. You provide us with no indication as to how far the patient should be able to walk, over what surface, and, for instance, if stair climbing is part of this evaluation.

SAMPLE SIZE

PRINCIPLE 110. JUSTIFY YOUR SAMPLE SIZE.

A description of the sample size calculations is a crucial, but often neglected part of the Methods section (Figures 23–5 and 23–6). When reviewing medical manuscripts, statistical consultants frequently ask the editor: "Can the authors provide any rationale or statistical power considerations underlying their choice of sample size?" (Colton 1990).

In addition, statisticians often ask: "Did the negative study have sufficient power to detect clinically meaningful effects, if such effects truly existed?" (Colton 1990).

Describe the method that you used to calculate the necessary sample size. Provide enough detail and adequate references so that others can reproduce your sample size calculations. Also reference the statistical book or software that you used.

PRINCIPLE 111. INTERPRET THE RESULTS OF SMALL STUDIES CAUTIOUSLY.

If your study has a small sample, discuss the low power of statistical tests. Do not include this interpretation of your sample size in the Methods section; it belongs in the Discussion. In studies with small samples, anticipate greater variance, lack of statistical power, and large differences that are not statistically significant, but nevertheless may be clinically important.

PRINCIPLE 112. DEMONSTRATE THAT YOU UNDERSTAND THE STATISTICAL POWER OF YOUR STUDY.

Describe the sample size that is necessary to achieve statistical significance, and provide a statistical basis for the number of patients included in your study. Although most clini-

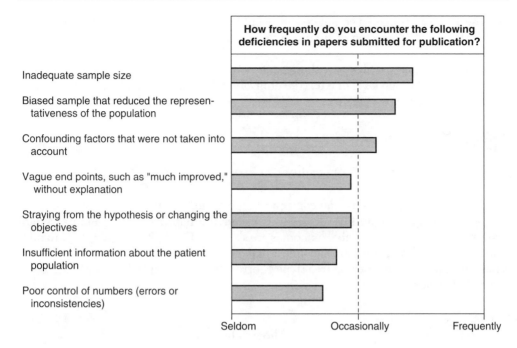

Figure 23–5. The frequency of research design problems. From question 23 of the Peer Review Questionnaire in Appendix B.

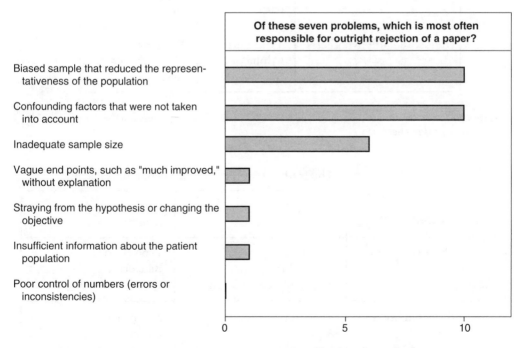

Figure 23–6. Research design problems and rejection. From question 24 of the Peer Review Questionnaire in Appendix B.

cal research papers need a complete statement about sample size, many do not include such a statement. These topics are discussed in more detail in Chapter 9.

To estimate sample size, begin with the standard power calculation settings: a power of 0.80 and a significance level of 0.05 (the equivalent of a 5% chance of a type I error and a 20% chance of a type II error).

⊕ FOR MORE INFORMATION

See Sample Size Software in Appendix D.

Many people are confused by the concept of type I and type II errors (Figure 23–7). A simple way to understand this idea is to consider the null hypothesis "innocent until proven guilty." The four possible outcomes are shown in Figure 23–8. A jury tries to minimize the possibility of convicting an innocent person (type I error) and minimize the possibility of setting a guilty person free (type II error). For each clinical research study, you too must balance the risk of these errors.

The null hypothesis is:

Decision	True	False
Accept the null hypothesis	No error (1 − alpha) 95%	Type II error (Beta) 20%
Reject the null hypothesis	Type I error (Alpha or *P*) 5%	No error (1 − beta, power) 80%

Figure 23–7. Illustration of type I and type II errors. The percentages represent the conventional levels that many researchers use.

The truth is that the assumption of innocence is:

The jury's verdict	True (Truly innocent)	False (Guilty)
Accept the assumption: Acquit	No error 1 − alpha Innocent person acquitted	Type II error Beta error Guilty person acquitted
Reject the assumption: Convict	Type I error Alpha error Innocent person convicted	No error Power Guilty person convicted

Figure 23–8. Analogy of a jury's decision illustrating type I and type II errors.

PRINCIPLE 113. Minimize the risk of a type I error.

Table 23–2 shows the features of a type I error.

PRINCIPLE 114. Minimize the risk of a type II error.

Table 23–3 shows the features of a type II error. In studies with small samples, report and discuss the power and probability of type II errors. Remember, type II errors are more common with small samples.

To remember these error types, use the following mnemonic device: A type I error is an alpha error, and A is the first letter of the alphabet. A type II error is a beta error, and B is the second letter of the alphabet. Then remember that alpha corresponds to the *P* value (typically 0.05).

PRINCIPLE 115. Report the median.

You can maximize the value of a small sample by using the data analysis techniques that professionals use. For example, you can report the median (middle value) rather than the mean for small samples, as well as for ordinal variables and for skewed data. In these situations, the median is a more accurate estimate of central tendency.

Example 23–4.

Group	Length of Stay (days)	Mean	Median
1	12, 12, **13,** 14, 14	13	13
2	12, 12, **13,** 14, 365	83	13

Example 23–4 shows that one number (365) distorts the mean, but not the median.

Table 23–2.   Features of a Type I Error

Rejection of a true null hypothesis
False claim of a difference
Common when a researcher is too ready to reject the null hypothesis
Alpha error
Occurs approximately 5% of the time with a P value threshold of <0.05
Analogous to convicting an innocent person

Table 23–3.   Features of a Type II Error

The chance of missing a real effect
An acceptance of a false null hypothesis
False claim of no difference when a difference actually exists, but the sample size is
    too small to prove it
Common when a researcher is too ready to accept the null hypothesis
Beta error
Occurs approximately 20% of the time with a power of 80% (power = $1 - \beta$)
Analogous to acquitting a guilty person

If you decide to report a median rather than a mean, report the median for similar variables throughout the paper. Mixing medians and means for similar variables may confuse readers and make them suspicious.

STATISTICAL ANALYSIS

PRINCIPLE 116. MAKE THE STATISTICS EASY TO UNDERSTAND.

Show that you understand the statistical methods used and can clearly report the statistical results. Although most reviewers are highly skilled physicians, many need help understanding the statistical analysis used in most modern studies.

Verify that the Methods section describes the statistical analysis adequately. The statistician and the primary writer must work together and should check the final draft to ensure that their sections fit together seamlessly. Inconsistencies in the description of the statistical analysis may raise questions about the quality of your work.

Example 23–5.

If, instead of writing "logistic regression," you write "logistical regression" or "logistics regression," reviewers may have trouble believing anything else that you say.

Describe exactly where (in your paper) and why you used the principal tests. In addition to using the correct tests, you must interpret each one adequately. If you used any unusual statistical methods, reference them and explain why you decided not to use more common statistical methods. You cannot simply say that you applied matching and logistic regression. Describe them in detail, and explain precisely how you used them.

◎ VITAL POINT

Edit the description of the statistical analysis carefully.

Many reviewers do not have the necessary skills to evaluate statistics. When editors were asked: "Do you feel that you have adequate skills to evaluate the statistical aspects of most medical manuscripts you are asked to review?," 29% of the editors said "No." In response to the same question, twice as many reviewers (58%) said "No." Although many of the editors said that they consulted statistical reviewers when necessary, you can help reviewers and editors by revising your description until you minimize the possibility of misinterpretation.

In summary, it is important to use the correct statistical tests and to recognize when your sample is too small; describing your statistical analysis in detail is every bit as important.

PRINCIPLE 117. DEFINE STATISTICAL SIGNIFICANCE INTELLIGENTLY.

Include the word "considered" in descriptions of statistical significance such as: "A P value of less than 0.05 was considered statistically significant."

PRINCIPLE 118. PROVIDE REPRODUCIBLE DETAILS OF YOUR STATISTICAL METHODS.

Any professional data analyst given a copy of your data should be able to verify your results after reading the Methods section. Use this criterion to determine how much detail to provide.

PRINCIPLE 119. JUSTIFY YOUR CHOICE OF STATISTICAL TESTS.

A common criticism of reviewers is inappropriate use of statistical tests by authors. Without a clear explanation showing that the appropriate statistical methods were applied, reviewers may ask:

 Who oversaw the statistics?

 Does a statistician agree that the proper tests were done?

Explain why you performed the statistical analysis with the tests you chose. For example: Did you choose the test because your data were not normally distributed? Was the test designed for matched samples? Were the variables skewed? **Study the histograms, and use Figure 16–1 as a general guide for choosing the correct test.**

Explain and justify any potentially confusing terms, such as "rank order." If you recently learned a new statistical method, however, do not explain it in detail in your paper. Residents in particular should avoid belaboring the obvious. As a rule, information that is available in textbooks should not be explained in a scientific paper.

PRINCIPLE 120. INCLUDE YOUR STATISTICAL RECIPE.

In the Methods section, describe your statistical analysis.

Example 23–6.

All analyses were performed according to the intention-to-treat principle. We used the chi-square test (without the Yates correction) and Fisher's exact test for categorical comparisons of data. Differences in the means of continuous measurements were tested by the Student's t-test and checked by the Mann-Whitney U test. Significant predictors in the univariate analysis were then included in a forward, stepwise multiple logistic-regression model to identify the most important risk factors for a recurrence; patients for whom relevant data were missing were excluded from the multivariate analyses (Hosmer and Lemeshow 1989). Cox proportional-hazards analysis was used to determine the relative contribution of various factors to the risk of a recurrence (Cox 1972). A P value of <0.05 was considered to indicate statistical significance; all tests were two-tailed. All statistical analyses were performed on a personal computer with the statistical package SPSS for Windows (Version 7.5, SPSS, Chicago).

This example shows a basic description of statistical methods. For many journals, an even more detailed description is appropriate. An important point to remember is that if you did not use the chi-square and Student's *t*-tests, justify your decision.

Occasionally, when researchers want to prove that one treatment is not different from another treatment, they choose statistical tests for which it is more difficult to obtain a *P* value of less than 0.05. Explain your reasons for choosing specific tests, or readers may think that you are trying to fool them. Many prominent journals now have a separate statistical review—all the more reason that your statistical recipe must be complete.

⊕ FOR MORE INFORMATION

See Figure 16–1.

Table 23–4.   Commonly Used Statistical Symbols and Abbreviations

Symbol or Abbreviation	Description	Universal Code (for symbols)
Greek		
α = alpha	Probability of a type I error, significance level, P value, typically $P < .05$, a present rejection level.	25
β = beta	Probability of a type II error, $1 -$ power, typically 0.20	26
μ = mu	Mean, average	36
π = pi	Population proportion or 3.1415	40
σ = sigma (lowercase)	Population standard deviation	42
σ^2 = sigma squared	Population variance, standard deviation squared	42
χ^2 = chi-square	Chi-square statistic	47
Σ = sigma (uppercase)	Sum	18
Φ = phi	Phi coefficient	21
English		
ANOVA	ANalysis Of VAriance	
CI	Confidence interval	
df	Degrees of freedom	
e	Base of the system of natural (Napierian) logarithms (e = 2.71828)	
F	Variance ratio (between groups ÷ within groups)	
H_O	Null hypothesis	
H_A	Alternative hypothesis	
∞	Infinity	
N	Number in entire population, sample or size of finite population	
n	Number in a subsample or subset	
NS	Not significant	
OR	Odds ratio	
P	Probability (range, 0–1)	
r	Pearson correlation coefficient (range, -1–$+1$)	
r^2	Pearson correlation coefficient squared	
RR	Relative risk	
r_s	Spearman's rank correlation coefficient	
R	Multiple correlation	
R^2	R squared, amount of variation explained, multiple correlation squared	
s	Standard deviation of a sample mean	

(continued)

Table 23–4. Commonly Used Statistical Symbols and Abbreviations (*continued*)	
s^2	Variance of a sample mean
SD	Standard deviation of a sample
SEM	Standard error of the mean
t	Student's *t*-test statistic
X	Raw score, population data
x	Raw score, sample data
$\overline{X}$	Arithmetic mean of a population
$\overline{x}$	Arithmetic mean of a sample
Z	Observation X in standard form, standard score, standard normal variate, standard normal variable or distribution

PRINCIPLE 121. LEARN STATISTICAL SHORTHAND.

Understanding common statistical symbols, acronyms, and abbreviations will help you to interpret medical literature and read statistical books (Table 23–4). Chapter 28 (principle 205) explains how to print Greek and other symbols with your computer.

CHAPTER 24.

Results

ORGANIZING THE RESULTS

PRINCIPLE 122. PRESENT YOUR RESULTS ENTHUSIASTICALLY.

Most scientists are excited about their results, but many do not convey this excitement and consequently write dull manuscripts.

Archimedes' reaction may have been extreme—yelling "Eureka!"—when he discovered how to measure the purity of gold. Yet, imparting this spirit of excitement, especially in the first few sentences of the Results, would improve most manuscripts.

After you analyze your data, reflect on what it means. Save your interpretation for the Discussion, but do not report results like a robot. Never start the Results with a page of number-heavy text. Instead, summarize similar types of numbers in tables, and invest the time to create reader-friendly graphs. As with the Methods, organize your material to make the Results easy to read.

Often the most logical way to present your Results is to tell your story in the chronological order in which you discovered the findings, but omit the details of your thought process. **Do not overstate the results or repeat in detail information that is given in the tables.** Instead, refer the reader to the tables, and shorten the text of the Results. Follow the logical order outlined in your study notes. Keep the Results as organized and as simple as possible.

Example 24–1.

Outcome was compared between Group I and Group II.

PRINCIPLE 123. PRESENT YOUR DATA IN A NATURAL ORDER.

If the order of discovery does not provide an appropriate presentation, consider organizing the Results sequentially from the patients' perspective (e.g., prepregnancy, antepartum, postpartum) or topically (e.g., maternal, fetal).

Inadequate presentation of the results is a common reason for outright rejection. To avoid this problem, verify that your results and follow-up data are unambiguous, complete, accurate, and presented logically.

Groom messy data before submission. For example, when the N changes, explain why. Provide the precise number of incomplete data sets rather than vague statements about missing data (e.g., "data were complete for most patients").

Never bewilder the reader with statistics. Instead, translate, summarize, and interpret the results of your analysis. Strive for clarity and brevity. Then obtain a second opinion to verify that the presentation of your results is adequate and well structured, and that your **rationale is not confused or contradictory.**

PRINCIPLE 124. START YOUR RESULTS SECTION WITH THE MAJOR POSITIVE FINDINGS.

Describe the sample early in the Results. In the first sentence, state how many patients met the inclusion criteria, then state what percentage died (or had the primary outcome under investigation). Although it is very important to explain which patients were excluded or dropped from the analysis, avoid starting with a long explanation of the various groups that were excluded. **Report negative associations at the end of the Results.**

◎ VITAL POINT

Include a table describing the study patients. This will reduce reviewers' concerns about bias between the groups and differences between your sample and larger populations.

Describe the base population at the hospital or clinic from which the study sample was drawn. Make it easy for the reader to understand baseline rates for preexisting conditions and diseases that patients may have had. Avoid the words "demographics" and "parameters." Instead, use "variables," "factors," or "characteristics." Provide sufficient information about the patient population to avoid comments such as the following:

 More information needs to be provided about the population from which this sample was taken. Were they all seen at one hospital? Does this hospital specialize in high-risk pregnancies? What percentage had maternal complications?

How does this patient population differ from published studies that have different conclusions? Table 1 should contain substance abuse, diabetes, hypertension, and so forth.

Example 24–2.

Patients randomized to Group I were not statistically different from patients in Group II in terms of age, hypertension, or smoking history.

PRESENTING STATISTICAL INFORMATION

PRINCIPLE 125. REPORT THE RELATIVE RISK AND 95% CONFIDENCE INTERVALS.

Relative risk is the ratio of the incidence of outcome in the exposed group to the incidence of outcome in the unexposed group. In addition to giving outcome percentage for each group, results are often more convincing when you report relative risk.

Example 24–3.

You could say: "The complication rate was higher in Group I than in Group II (6.8% versus 1.7%)." However, reporting that "the complication rate was four times higher (relative risk 4.0, 95% confidence interval 2.1–6.1)" is more convincing.

The *odds ratio* measures the odds of having the risk factor among people with the disease divided by the odds of having the risk factor among people without the disease.

The odds ratio is typically used for case–control studies. Relative risk, incidence, and prevalence usually are not appropriate for case–control studies because the samples are not representative of the larger population.

Example 24–4.

A case–control study might compare 100 Vietnam veterans who attempted suicide with 100 Vietnam veterans who did not attempt suicide. Obviously, it would be wrong to conclude that 50% of Vietnam veterans attempt suicide. Similar problems occur when measures designed for population-based data are inappropriately used in case–control studies.

⊕ FOR MORE INFORMATION

For more details, see Fleiss (1981), Hulley and Cummings (1988), Kuzma (1992), and Sackett et al. (1991).

A 95% confidence interval for the relative risk is crucial. This interval shows readers the limits for which you can be assured with 95% confidence of the true relative risk for the study population (Figure 24–1). Provide confidence intervals for every relative risk and odds ratio. Never overestimate the size of an effect by providing only the relative risk without the confidence interval.

Critical readers will want to know whether the 95% confidence intervals include the value 1.0, and if not, how far they are from 1.0. A relative risk of 1.0 suggests there is no difference in the proportion of people with the disease between the exposed and the unexposed groups. A relative risk may be much higher than 1.0, but if the 95% confidence interval overlaps 1.0, you usually can conclude that the increase in risk is not statistically significant.

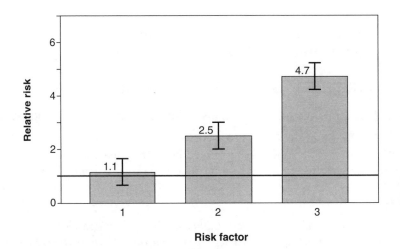

Figure 24–1. Example of the relative risk (RR) and 95% confidence intervals (CI) for three risk factors. For risk factor 1, the RR is greater than 1, but the 95% CI (the I-shaped symbol) clearly crosses the line. Therefore, you would conclude that risk factor 1 is not a significant factor (assuming that you had sufficient statistical power). Risk factors 2 and 3 have RR and CI values that clearly are greater than 1. Therefore, you would conclude that they are statistically significant risk factors.

When one group has no patients with the outcome under study, the exact relative risk cannot be calculated. In this case, report it as infinity (∞) with confidence intervals, as in the following example.

Example 24–5.

Relative risk = ∞; 95% confidence interval = 4.7 to ∞.

In summary, always provide confidence intervals for your primary results. Adding confidence intervals improves most papers, and these values can be calculated easily with most statistical packages. Be aware, however, that authors sometimes divide the wrong percentages, so verify that you have calculated the relative risk correctly (Figure 24–2).

⊕ FOR MORE INFORMATION

See Dawson-Saunders and Trapp (1994); Kleinbaum, Kupper, and Morgenstern (1982); and Mehta, Patel, and Gray (1985). Gardner and Altman (1989) have written an excellent book on confidence intervals: *Statistics with Confidence.*

PRINCIPLE 126. USE STATISTICAL TERMS SKILLFULLY.

1. **Significant** means "probably caused by something other than mere chance." Medical researchers customarily label findings "statistically significant" if the probability of their finding occurring by chance is less than 5% ($P < 0.05$). Verify that your Results show statistically significant findings when you use the word "significant." Otherwise,

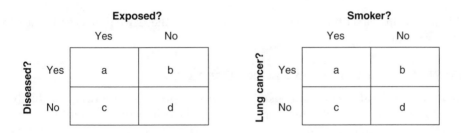

		a / (a+c)	Incidence among exposed persons
Relative risk		b / (b+d)	Incidence among nonexposed persons
Attributable risk		$\left(a / (a+c)\right) - \left(b / (b+d)\right)$	Incidence among exposed persons – Incidence among nonexposed persons
Odds ratio (relative odds)		$\dfrac{ad}{cb}$ or $\dfrac{a/b}{c/d}$	Odds that diseased person was exposed to risk factor Odds that nondiseased person was exposed to risk factor

Figure 24–2. Relative risk, attributable risk, and odds ratio.

later in the Discussion, clarify what may be clinically significant despite the lack of statistical significance, especially with small samples.

Reviewers may be confused and say:

> For Figure 2, no P values are displayed, nor are they in the legend, even though there is a statement about "significant differences."

2. **Random** refers to the idea that each element in a set has an equal probability of occurrence. Do not use the word "random" to mean "haphazard," "unplanned," or "incidental."
3. A **sample** is "a finite part of a statistical population whose properties are studied to gain information about the whole" (*Merriam-Webster's Collegiate Dictionary* 1993). "Sample" has this technical meaning in research. Other uses of the term only confuse the reader.
4. A **random sample** is a chance selection in which all members of the base population presumably have the same chance of being selected. Random sampling is commonly used to reduce bias.
5. **Correlation** is a statistical measure of the strength of the linear relationship between two continuous variables. The term "correlation" should not be used in a nonstatistical sense, especially in a title. Do not describe the association between categorical variables as a "correlation." **Use "correlation" only with two interval-level variables.** For example, if you report a correlation with race, reviewers may think that you are mathematically illiterate. Also, when you report the results of a correlation, never confuse the correlation coefficient (r) with R squared (R^2), which is a regression statistic.

Ambiguous technical writing annoys reviewers, so avoid these five pitfalls and be alert for similar problems.

PRINCIPLE 127. PRESENT P VALUES PROFESSIONALLY.

Provide exact P values. Do not use "NS" (not significant) or inequalities (e.g., $P < 0.05$). Before personal computers permitted the calculation of exact P values, researchers often were forced to use these vague terms. Researchers looked up the critical values for their sample size in statistics textbooks. These tables provided rough estimates of P values (< 0.05 or < 0.01). Avoid this outdated method of reporting P values.

In the following situations, however, you cannot or should not use an exact P value.

- If the P value is less than 0.001, report "$P < 0.001$." Do not report "$P = 0.000006$."
- If the P value is nearly 1.0, some software packages report "$P > 0.95$"; this terminology is acceptable.
- Multiple comparison tests often do not provide exact P values, but show inequalities (e.g., "$P < 0.05$").

Use a consistent number of decimal places to report P values. For example, do not report "$P < 0.1$" in one place and "$P < 0.00005$" in another. The use of three places ordinarily is sufficient (e.g., $P = 0.024$, $P < 0.001$). Provide P values for variables in tables, even if the comparison is 0% versus 0%. Use a program (e.g., True Epistat; see Appendix D) to double check all P values in the final draft of your manuscript. Explain any discrepancies, or reviewers may tell you:

> The P value of 0.1 on line 7 of page 10 should be checked. According to my calculations, the P value is 0.218.

Do not report P values without other pertinent information (e.g., mean, standard deviation, confidence interval). In the Results section, qualify P values and significance with the statistical test used. Avoid orphaned P values by stating which statistical tests you selected to compute each P value. An orphaned P value is presented without indication of the statistical test used. In the footnotes for tables, specify which statistical tests were used to compute which P values. Never imply significance when none exists.

Finally, do not use the standard error of the mean (SEM) in place of the standard deviation (SD) to mislead readers into believing that the variability is small. Remember that the SEM is calculated by dividing the SD by the square root of the sample size (n). The standard error of the mean is used to estimate the precision of the larger population mean from the sample mean.

⊕ FOR MORE INFORMATION

To learn more about the differences between the standard deviation and the standard error of the mean, see Bartko (1985).

PRINCIPLE 128. INTERPRET P VALUES INTELLIGENTLY.

Avoid saying that a small P value proves that your findings are strong. A weak association or a small difference also can produce a small P value. Consider evidence beyond the P value. Use your clinical judgment to evaluate the magnitude and importance of differences. On the other hand, do not dismiss differences between study groups that fall within the normal range.

⊕ FOR MORE INFORMATION

See Bailar and Mosteller (1992); Salsburg (1985); Ware, Mosteller, and Ingelfinger (1992); and Yancey (1990).

ANTICIPATING PITFALLS IN THE RESULTS

PRINCIPLE 129. REPORT RESULTS IN THE TARGET JOURNAL'S FORMAT.

For some journals, especially psychology and psychiatry journals, you must be sure to report the degrees of freedom and the statistic's test value. To speed the submission and review process, include this information in your first draft. The *Publication Manual of the American Psychological Association* (APA 1994) describes the required format in great detail.

Example 24–6.

The rate of depression was higher in Group I than in Group II, $\chi^2(1, N = 200) = 11.31$, p < .05.

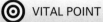 VITAL POINT

Even if the target journal does not require this level of detail, keep all important statistical printouts organized in a binder because you may have to submit your paper to another journal that does.

Keep a copy of the data file (database or spreadsheet) and the system file for the statistical package on a diskette. Label, document, and organize this material because you may need it years later. For example, an editor may agree to publish your paper if you add the degrees of freedom and the statistic's test values. In this situation, you will need to refer to the statistical printouts.

The following is an overview of degrees of freedom. *Degrees of freedom (df)* is a concept used in statistics to determine the most appropriate distribution for calculating the *P* value for your sample size and number of groups. For the chi-square, you can calculate the degrees of freedom as follows:

(Number of rows − 1) × (Number of columns − 1)

Example 24–7.

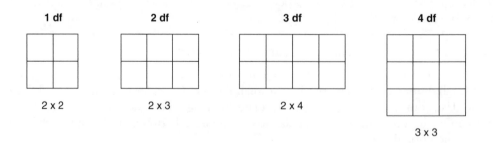

For the Student's *t*-test (using the pooled variance method), calculate the degrees of freedom by subtracting 2 from the total sample size (*df* = n − 2).

PRINCIPLE 130. DESCRIBE PEOPLE SENSITIVELY AND DIPLOMATICALLY.

When you describe people in your study, avoid all potentially pejorative terms. Providing a general guideline for this principle is impossible, but Table 24–1 shows examples.

During the course of your study, especially during data cleaning and analysis, you can protect the confidentiality of patients by using case numbers rather than names. However, in your paper, **be sensitive about using the word "cases" to describe people.** Describe the person first, and then name the disease or disability. **"Patients with diabetes" is appropriate; "people of smoke" is a bit extreme.** Table 24–2 shows diplomatic terms that can be used.

Table 24–1. Pejorative Terms to Avoid

Pejorative Term	*Preferred Term*
Wheelchair-bound people	Persons who use wheelchairs
Mental disorders	Impaired cognitive function
Mentally ill person	Person with mental illness
SCI patients versus normal patients	Person with spinal cord injury versus able-bodied persons
Diabetic pregnancies	Pregnancies complicated by diabetes
Four of the five recurrences died	Four of the five patients with recurrences died.
Among elective THR patients	Among patients who undergo elective THR
Of THR patients	Of patients who have undergone THR
Elective THR patients, patients with total hip arthroplasty	Patients who underwent THR
In 43 patients used as controls	For 43 patients who served as controls
Schizophrenics	People diagnosed with schizophrenia
Epileptics	People with epilepsy
The elderly	Older people

Table 24–2. Diplomatic Terms to Use

Problematic Term	*Preferred Term*
Subject, individual, case, patient (in some cases)	Respondent, man, woman, subject, participant
45 males	45 male patients, 45 men
67 females	67 female patients, 67 women
Chairman	Chairperson, chair
Managing patients	Treating patients
Patients who developed X	Patients in whom X developed
Two patients developed X	Two patients had X
Had surgery	Underwent surgery
Few mortalities	Few deaths
Demise	Death
Expired, succumbed	Died
Primary procedures accounted for 87 patients.	Primary procedures were performed on 87 patients.
Patients have worse outcome	Patients experience worse outcome
Patients with complications	Patients who experience complications
None of the 27 patients had a complication.	No complications occurred in the 27 patients.
Had a complication	Experienced a complication
Patients with extended hospitalizations	Patients who stayed in the hospital for extended periods
Fetus was aborted	Pregnancy was terminated

(continued)

Table 24–2. Diplomatic Terms to Use (*continued*)	
Cesarean section, c-section	Cesarean delivery
Cesarean section for fetal distress	Fetal risk requiring cesarean delivery
Intrauterine growth retardation	Intrauterine growth restriction
Motor vehicle accidents	Motor vehicle collisions
Accidents in the home	Injuries in the home
Man and wife	Husband and wife, man and woman
Orientals	Asian people
Senility	Dementia

PRINCIPLE 131. Write a comprehensive and convincing Results section.

In many papers, the Results section is too short (see Figure 12–1). Do not limit the Results to a few variables significantly related to the primary outcome.

Provide results for the most severe form of outcome. For example, describe the mortality rate overall and for important subgroups. Although it is impossible to define the appropriate length for all papers, if your paper has less than two double-spaced pages of Results, you probably should add more findings before you submit it. If you are not sure what to add, try to anticipate which results researchers will need to include in their meta-analysis.

Show the consistency of your evidence from different angles, or you may give the impression that your **data are inconclusive: a common reason for rejection.**

Example 24–8.

If you found an association between alcohol use and a certain outcome, do not rely on one P value to convince readers. Analyze drinks per day, drink-years, and subgroups (e.g., nonsmokers).

For more information about the consistency of evidence, see principle 134.

Especially when reporting the outcome of different treatments, make it easy for the reader to understand that you controlled for the severity of disease. Explain which variables you controlled for, and how. Although some of this information is included in your Methods, the Results must show that your methods of controlling for confounding factors actually worked. Provide separate results for patients with a good prognosis and those with a poor prognosis. Report results for patients who underwent primary surgery separately from results for those who underwent revisions. If you omit or ignore important data, reviewers may ask for additional details. For example:

 How many women with gestational diabetes required insulin therapy?

If the Results section is too long, reviewers may say:

My only criticism is that the Results section is entirely too long, especially given the completeness of the tables. It should be rewritten for brevity.

 The results are reported in elaborate detail. In my opinion, the description of the results in the text is far too long—much of the content of pages 12 to 17 simply elaborates on what is in the tables. The same information could be conveyed much more economically.

However, in most rejected manuscripts, the Results section is too short (see Figure 12–1). If two pages of Results are all you have, do another literature search and then re-analyze your data to compare with published results. Finally, never write a Results section that leaves the reader with the impression of overanalysis or data dredging. By chance alone, 1 in every 20 statistical tests will provide a P value of < 0.05. For this reason, reviewers may be concerned that your findings are the result of testing too many variables.

◎ VITAL POINT

Make a long Results section easier to read by including subheadings.

PRINCIPLE 132. ACKNOWLEDGE THAT YOU ARE AWARE OF SMALL CELL SIZES.

Some subgroups presented in the text and tables may be too small to permit any sensible analysis. Combine the categories into cells with larger N values, or explain your reasons for not doing so.

Example 24–9.

In an analysis of pressure ulcer patients grouped by anatomic level of spinal cord injury, certain subgroups may contain few patients. However, for some readers, knowing the number of patients with a lesion at each level may be important. Combining injuries into general categories (e.g., cervical, thoracic, lumbar) would make it impossible for these readers to get the information they need.

In situations such as this one, you can report the results using specific categories and then combine them for statistical analysis when needed. Always record information in as much detail as possible, and then, if necessary, combine the values into more general categories for analysis.

PRINCIPLE 133. SPECIFY A FOLLOW-UP TIME FRAME WHEN REPORTING RATES.

Example 24–10.

Stating that "the recurrence rate of pressure ulcers was 17%" is meaningless without an explicitly defined follow-up period. Instead, state that "during the first postoperative year, the recurrence rate of pressure ulcers was 14.2%."

To calculate a true rate, you need three pieces of information:

1. The number of patients with the study condition
2. The size of the population at risk
3. A time frame

Researchers most often forget to include the third piece of information: a time frame. Table 24–3 shows three examples of rate calculations.

⊕ FOR MORE INFORMATION

See Mausner and Kramer (1985).

PRINCIPLE 134. USE THE TOOLS OF PROFESSIONAL EPIDEMIOLOGISTS TO EVALUATE AND REPORT CAUSATION.

Many clinical research papers that evaluate cause and effect can be improved by applying the criteria shown in Table 24–4.

⊕ FOR MORE INFORMATION

See Hill (1965); Kleinbaum, Kupper, and Morgenstern (1982); Mausner and Kramer (1985); Rothman (1986); and Sackett et al. (1991).

Table 24–3.   Formulas for Calculating Rates

$$\text{Rate} = \frac{\text{Outcomes during a specific period}}{\text{Population at risk for the outcome during a specific period}}$$

$$\text{Attack rate} = \frac{\text{Number of persons ill during a specific period}}{\text{Number of persons at risk during a specific period}}$$

$$\text{Neonatal mortality rate} = \frac{\text{Number of deaths of liveborn infants (0 to 27 days of age) in a year}}{\text{Number of live births in the same year}}$$

Table 24–4.   Criteria for Evaluating Causation

Strength of the study design
Strength of the association (usually a statistic, such as a relative risk of 18.4 or r = 0.782)
Dose–response relationship
Temporally correct association
Consistency of the findings (from different studies)
Biologic plausibility of the hypothesis (consistency with existing knowledge)
Specificity of the association (predictive value)

Table 24–5. Criteria for Evaluating a Clinical Scale
Consistent statistical evidence from the data in support of each factor
Biologically plausible interpretation for the causal mechanism underlying each factor
Evidence in the literature that each factor was associated with the development of the outcome
Improvement in the sensitivity and specificity of the total score caused by the addition of each factor

PRINCIPLE 135. USE RIGOROUS SCIENTIFIC METHODS TO CREATE A NEW CLINICAL SCALE OR PREDICTIVE INDEX.

A *clinical scale* usually is a simple scoring system designed to help health care professionals estimate the risk that an outcome will occur. The criteria shown in Table 24–5 can help you to design a quality scale.

⊕ FOR MORE INFORMATION

See Dawson-Saunders and Trapp (1994) and Sackett et al. (1991). For an example of a paper that presents a new scale, see Salzberg et al. (1996).

PRINCIPLE 136. MAKE CLEAR WHAT WAS ADJUSTED FOR WITH YOUR MULTIVARIATE ANALYSIS.

When you present the results of multivariate analysis, explain which factors were controlled for in the model. Although you may have described the analysis in the Methods, in your Results, explain which tests were used. Do not make broad statements (e.g., "After adjusting for preoperative factors . . ."). And for regression models, report the goodness of fit.

PRINCIPLE 137. PRESENT NUMBERS FOR SIMILAR VARIABLES CONSISTENTLY.

Use a consistent number of decimal places. As a rule, use one decimal place for the mean and standard deviation of whole numbers.

Example 24–11.

The mean age in Group I was significantly lower than that in Group II (42.7 ± 3.3 versus 53.8 ± 2.6, P = 0.014).

Of course, consult the target journal's instructions for authors and recent issues of the target journal to identify any deviations from these guidelines, but never report numbers to meaningless decimal places (e.g., the average venous pH was 7.42179, the mean age was 27.21 years).

PRINCIPLE 138. INCLUDE ONLY RESULTS IN THE RESULTS SECTION.

Focus on your hypothesis, and move any interpretations of the results to the Discussion. Separate the Results and the Discussion—completely. For example, the following sentence is an interpretation and should be moved to the Discussion: "This finding is not entirely unexpected."

◎ VITAL POINT

The Results section rarely requires references. A sentence that requires a reference probably belongs in another section.

Sometimes investigators expect to find certain results, but the data do not agree with their preconceived notions. **Describe** this situation at the end of the Results, but **discuss** it in the Discussion section. These negative findings certainly will interest many of your peers.

TABLES

PRINCIPLE 139. DESIGN READER-FRIENDLY TABLES.

Well-designed tables and figures are more important than most medical researchers realize because reviewers often read them first. As with your title and abstract, make a good first impression with your tables, but remember that editors often object to the inclusion of more than a few tables; redundant tables and graphs add unnecessary length and cost.

◎ VITAL POINT

Do not include more than the average number of tables or graphs for the target journal.

Many readers have trouble interpreting tables, so make your tables clear and focused. Anticipate how the reader will mentally sort rows, and consider revising your table to reflect that order.

In tables, include only pertinent data, and avoid redundancies. A person who skips the text and reads only your tables should be able to draw conclusions similar to yours.

Often, you can make your tables easier to read by adding the percentage for each row.

Example 24–12.

Tables often show the column percentage of men and women, forcing readers to mentally calculate the row percentage for the mortality rates among men and among women.

	Survived (n = 870)	Died (n = 63)	Row Percentage	P Value
Sex				< 0.001
Male	22.1%	42.9%	12.3%	
Female	77.9%	57.1%	5.0%	

Remember, you can improve your tables by considering the ordering and calculations that readers would perform mentally.

PRINCIPLE 140. DO NOT REPEAT INFORMATION IN THE TABLES AND TEXT.

Many writers repeat information in the text and tables. This mistake irritates both re-viewers and editors. Make sure, however, that the text agrees with the tables and figures.

For example, are the inclusion criteria inconsistent between the Methods and the tables? If so, verify that the data are correct, and add a footnote to the table to explain why the information is correct, but appears inconsistent.

Explain any significant differences between the tables and the text. Describe the medical diagnoses in the text or a table, but not both.

Avoid abbreviations in tables. If you must use abbreviations (e.g., to save space), **define each one** in the table's footnotes.

Explain in the text the numbers in the tables. If the number of subjects changes, explain the change. **If some patients have more than one condition, add a footnote to the table explaining why the percentages do not total properly.** Keep the tables sim-ple, but not informal. For example, all tables need column headings.

PRINCIPLE 141. CREATE HIGH-QUALITY TABLES.

Table 24–6 shows a checklist of the components of a quality table.

PRINCIPLE 142. CITE AND SUMMARIZE ALL TABLES AND FIGURES IN THE TEXT.

Many reviewers highlight the citation for each table and figure in the text (e.g., "see Table 1") to verify that all citations are complete. In the text of the Results, emphasize the key point of each table and graph.

Remember to place the tables, figures, and figure legends after the text and the refer-ences.

PRINCIPLE 143. PRESENT ADVERSE OUTCOMES PERCEPTIVELY.

Report all complications and side effects objectively and in detail. Comparing complication rates between study groups requires thoughtful analysis and organization. In some reports, investigators attempt to obscure the truth by overwhelming the reader with tables of re-

---

Table 24–6.   Checklist for Creating a Table

- ✔ Simple and self-explanatory
- ✔ Format for the target journal followed
- ✔ Not a repetition of the text
- ✔ Double-spaced
- ✔ Units provided for each variable
- ✔ ± Values identified as either a standard deviation or a standard error of the mean
- ✔ Exact *P* values included
- ✔ Values rounded appropriately
- ✔ Format consistent with the other tables
- ✔ No vertical lines

sults. However, if you want to publish your findings, remember that reviewers expect a realistic comparison to answer the question: Do the benefits outweigh the adverse effects of this treatment? Complex tables are not a substitute for intelligent analysis of the findings.

Reviewers expect an accurate and honest account of the side effects of therapy in your study population and the limits of follow-up for side effects.

If your study was not a randomized clinical trial, be careful when you interpret data or outcome as "caused by" different therapies. Causality is difficult to prove for many reasons. Treatment protocols change over time, and patients with more severe disease often are given more aggressive treatment (or combinations of treatment) than patients with less severe disease. If your study was not designed to compare treatments and yet shows differences in outcome for different treatment groups, you have two choices:

1. Do not focus on the outcome analysis.
2. State the limitations of your interpretations, and describe the indications for each treatment.

PRINCIPLE 144. ADD A SIMPLE TABLE TO SOLVE ANTICIPATED CRITICISMS.

If your paper does not have too many tables, adding a table may make it easier for the reviewer to understand your conclusions. Ask yourself: **Would another table or graph avoid any anticipated criticism or confusion?** If your manuscript has more tables than average, you may be able to combine some of the information into a summary table.

PRINCIPLE 145. GIVE THE READER AMPLE RESULTS IN TABLES.

To convince readers of the validity of your claims, provide adequate data in the tables. For small studies, provide raw data for readers to analyze. Consider using a table of the key variables for each subject, but never include the patients' initials. Using a table will avoid the following type of comment:

 With only 20 patients, a table of the raw data for the most important variables would enable the reader to verify these findings.

Sometimes a table can show that the poor outcome in one group was caused specifically by the problem under study. You can use a table that stratifies patients into subgroups or one that presents the results of the multivariate analysis.

You can help the reader by providing not only the number of patients, but also the number of hospitals, observers, clinicians, and days of follow-up. You can provide this information in the text or tables of the Results.

FIGURES

PRINCIPLE 146. USE GRAPHS AND OTHER FIGURES TO ILLUSTRATE THE MAJOR POINTS.

Visual displays can help readers to understand your findings. Many readers prefer to look at a graph rather than a page of numbers or text. Consider using a variety of types of figures (e.g., graphs, diagrams, flowcharts, computer displays, photographs, radiographs, micrographs, anatomic drawings, family trees) to illustrate different points. Anticipate what reviewers might prefer to see in a graph:

 A bar graph for the comparisons on pages 9 and 10 would make it much easier to understand the differences among the groups.

◎ VITAL POINT

Use graphs to illustrate only the major points, particularly those that cannot easily be expressed in the text or tables.

A three-dimensional graph that shows the results of multivariate analysis is a perfect example of this point. A pie graph that shows the percentage of men and women included in a study is the mark of an amateur. As with tables, figures should agree with, but not repeat, information in the text. If you include superfluous or repetitive figures, reviewers may respond as follows:

 Neither Figure 1 nor Figure 2 is needed.

 I do not think that illustrations 6 and 7 add anything, and they should be omitted.

For each figure, ask yourself: Would a table present this finding more clearly? Figures show trends and multiple comparisons more effectively than tables. Tables are more effective for presenting a mixture of variables that cannot be displayed on the same scale.

Ask a colleague who is experienced in creating medical graphs to review your paper and tables and suggest better ways to graph the major points.

If you have several graphs with the same horizontal axis label, you often can combine them into one figure by stacking them. This technique helps the reader and allows you to use more graphs without exceeding the limit.

PRINCIPLE 147. CREATE PROFESSIONAL FIGURE LEGENDS.

Provide a detailed, easy-to-understand legend for each figure that clearly explains each graphic symbol. Again, avoid abbreviations. Check the accuracy of all figures—twice. Obviously, all information should be completely translated into English or omitted.

◎ VITAL POINT

Obtain written permission for any figures or tables that you borrow from published work.

PRINCIPLE 148. PAY ATTENTION TO DETAILS.

Label each axis clearly. For example, the Y-axis label should be perpendicular to the text and parallel to the Y-axis. Use thick lines and text that is large enough to read when the figure is reduced to fit on a journal page. When your graph is reduced to fit in a column, the axis labels should be similar in size to the printed text. You can reduce your graph on a photocopier to see how it will look. Edit the graph until it is as uncluttered and professional as possible. Use the *New England Journal of Medicine* as a guide.

Use a sans serif typeface (e.g., Helvetica), and do not automatically accept the defaults in your graphics software package. For example, software packages often will place legends in inappropriate places; move them as necessary.

Avoid imposing three-dimensional effects on two-dimensional bar and line graphs. Graphs created on a personal computer often are cluttered with background lines and too many axis numbers. Delete all unnecessary lines and numbers.

For each graph, identify the number of patients in each subgroup. For example, in each bar graph, each bar should indicate the number of cases (e.g., 9/17). Use "No. of patients" rather than "# patients." Each bar also should have a percentage to help the reader understand the point of the figure. In addition, clearly indicate the overall sample size for the graph.

Finally, never attach glossy prints with paper clips.

PRINCIPLE 149. EDIT OR REDESIGN SLIDE GRAPHS BEFORE YOU INCLUDE THEM IN YOUR MANUSCRIPT.

Do not submit prints of your slides as substitutes for professionally prepared tables or figures. The text of an oral presentation is much different from the text of a paper for publication. If you are writing a paper based on a slide presentation, do not attempt to include all of the presentation slides as graphs.

⊕ FOR MORE INFORMATION

If you have trouble with graphs, figures, slides, or conference posters, seek help from a professional. For glossy prints, slides, and posters, you will need a professional and reliable commercial photography lab. I rely on Spectratone Color Labs (see Appendix D). If you need a referral, the Association of Medical Illustrators can recommend a freelance medical artist or photographer (see Appendix D). See the Medical Illustrators home page on the Internet for samples. Briscoe's (1996) book *Preparing Scientific Illustrations* is also a good source for more information.

PRINCIPLE 150. USE FLOWCHARTS TO MAKE CLINICAL TRIALS EASY TO UNDERSTAND.

A flowchart is a diagram of boxes and connecting lines that shows the steps in a system, such as a study protocol. For randomized clinical trials, you can use a flowchart to illustrate the number of patients at each stage and in each arm or branch of the study. One flowchart often can replace a drab page of text in your Results. A good flowchart provides a clear picture of the patients at each phase. See Ewigman et al. (1995) for an example of how effective a flowchart can be.

Because many reviewers like to sketch out a flowchart as they read, anticipate this need. Providing a flowchart will make it easier for reviewers to read your paper. If you leave it up to reviewers to create their own flowcharts, they may become annoyed if their numbers do not agree with yours. Flowcharts also can illustrate the study protocol, testing scheme, and pattern of decisions.

PRINCIPLE 151. USE SCATTERGRAMS TO INTERPRET AND DISPLAY THE DISTRIBUTION OF TWO CONTINUOUS VARIABLES.

A scattergram, also called a "scatter diagram," a "scatterplot," or an "X-Y graph," is a two-dimensional graph of two continuous variables (Figure 24–3). A scattergram of the results can help you to identify more appropriate ways to analyze the data. You can use statistical software to create scattergrams quickly so that you can examine the data visually.

Consider including a scattergram of the primary point in your paper. Plot the individual points (with one continuous variable on the X-axis and the other on the Y-axis) to show the distribution of the individual points and how they fit a regression line. Use different symbols to identify the groups. Any superimposed points must be marked in some way, or a reviewer may count the points on the scattergram and complain about any discrepancies.

To create high-quality figures for publication, transfer your data to a graphics package (e.g., Freelance Graphics by the Lotus division of IBM or PowerPoint by Microsoft). You can edit these graphs to produce a professional image. Then you can print the edited graph on a laser printer (in high resolution) and take the final version to a photographer to be made into a black and white, 5- $\times$ 7-inch or 8- $\times$ 10-inch glossy print.

◎ VITAL POINT

When your results differ from published studies, try to create graphs and tables similar in format to those that have been published to make it easier for readers to compare them. Interpret your graphs with an open mind. Ask yourself what the authors of the contradicting studies would conclude from your graphs.

PRINCIPLE 152. USE HISTOGRAMS OR POLYGONS TO AID YOUR CHARACTERIZATION OF KEY DISTRIBUTIONS.

For the most important continuous variable in your study, explain the histogram's distribution in the text of the Results. For example, is it normal or skewed? If it is skewed, how severely is it skewed, and in which direction? Is it bimodal? Figure 24–4 shows an example of bimodal data.

PRINCIPLE 153. BE CREATIVE, AND USE GRAPHS TO COMMUNICATE MORE EFFECTIVELY.

You can use a cumulative frequency polygon, a stacked bar graph, a true three-dimensional graph (not just a three-dimensional effect), or a graph that illustrates the relative change from the control group. Scan top journals to get fresh ideas. Keep in mind that some journals now encourage the use of color in figures.

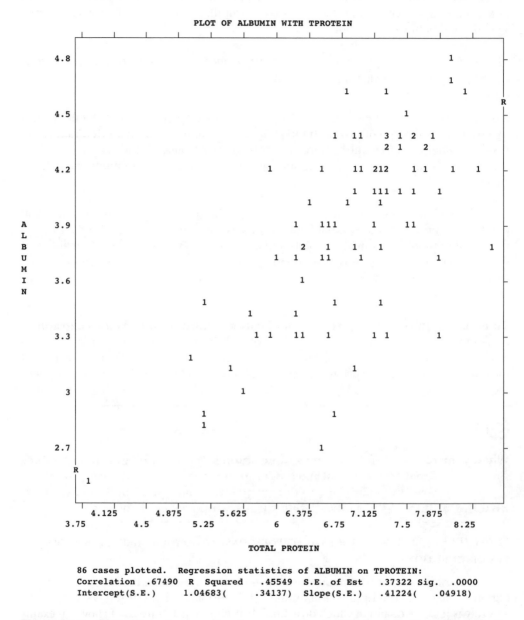

Figure 24–3. Scattergram of serum albumin concentration and total protein. The numbers in the graph are superimposed points. If you connect the R on the left with the R on the right, you would obtain a regression line. These results could be reported as follows: "Serum albumin was significantly correlated with total protein (r = 0.67, P < 0.001)."

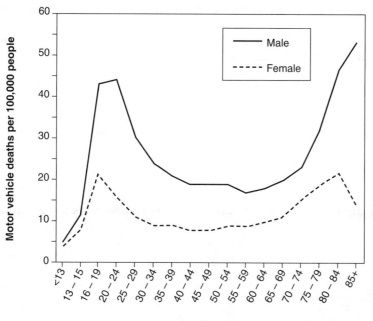

Figure 24–4. Polygon of bimodal data. Adapted from the Status Report of the Insurance Institute for Highway Safety. Vol. 30. Arlington (VA): Insurance Institute for Highway Safety; August 12, 1995.

⊕ FOR MORE INFORMATION

See Briscoe (1996).

PRINCIPLE 154. DISPLAY THE NORMAL RANGE AS BACKGROUND FOR LABORATORY AND CLINICAL DATA.

For major findings, especially the results of laboratory tests, provide the normal values. When you graph your findings, add the normal range (e.g., shaded as a band in the background). Providing a normal range specific to the study population is even better.

PRINCIPLE 155. GRAPH NEW CUTOFF POINTS ON AN ROC CURVE.

Receiver operator characteristics (ROC) curves are useful for selecting the most appropriate cutoff point for screening tests. On the Y-axis, plot the sensitivity. On the X-axis, plot the value that is 100 minus the specificity. Calculate the sensitivity and specificity at various cutoff points, and connect the points with a line. Draw a diagonal line from the top left corner to the bottom right corner. The intersection of this diagonal line with the curved plotted line provides an objective cutoff point. Be sure that your graph has a frame that is square, not rectangular. You usually can see the "elbow" of the line clearly as the point that is closest to the upper left corner.

Whenever you suggest a new cutoff point, provide an ROC curve. Show that you examined the data carefully to determine this new cutoff point. Include sufficient raw data to show that you chose the single best cutoff point. Do not expect anyone to take your word for this type of finding.

Several alternatives to the ROC curve are available:

- Create a graph with two lines (one for sensitivity and one for specificity), with various cutoff points along the X-axis. You can use the point at which these lines intersect to estimate the most appropriate cutoff point.
- Create a bar graph comparing two means, including 95% confidence intervals. Assuming that the good outcome group has a higher mean, you can use the lower limit of the 95% confidence interval for the group with good outcome to estimate the best cutoff point.
- To display a new cutoff point with this method, use two vertical bars comparing the means. **Add the 95% confidence intervals as I-shaped lines for each bar.** You can use a one-way analysis of variance (ANOVA) on a statistical package to calculate the 95% confidence intervals. For this type of graph, the 95% confidence intervals usually are more appropriate than the standard deviation or the standard error of the mean.

⊕ FOR MORE INFORMATION

See Fletcher, Fletcher, and Wagner (1996) and Sackett et al. (1991).

PRINCIPLE 156. KEEP GRAPHS SIMPLE, BUT SCIENTIFIC.

Make your graphs eye-catching, but simple. On the other hand, do not eliminate important details. For example, for survival curves, include the number of patients at risk during each interval of follow-up, and indicate that the scale reflects probability, not actual percentage of outcome.

PRINCIPLE 157. DISTINGUISH AMONG "PERCENT," "PERCENTAGE," AND "PERCENTILE."

When you graph a change, be sure that you understand the meanings of the terms "percent," "percentage," and "percentile." A change from 80% to 40% is a decrease of 40 percentage points, but a 50 percent decrease. Unless it appears in a table's column heading,

---

Table 24–7.   Checklist for Creating a Figure
✔ Thick lines
✔ Large text
✔ Exact *P* values
✔ Clear, detailed legend
✔ Information that is not included in the text
✔ Numbers displayed for each subgroup
✔ Easy-to-understand axis labels
✔ Meaningful use of shading and cross-hatching
✔ Self-explanatory

"percent" usually is preceded by a number (e.g., 20.7 percent, 100 percent). Otherwise, use "percentage" (e.g., "A large percentage of patients . . ."). "Percent" is not used as a noun in most medical writing.

Percentile is "a value on a scale of one hundred that indicates the percent of a distribution that is equal to or below it (a score in the 95th percentile)" (*Merriam-Webster's Collegiate Dictionary* 1993).

⊕ FOR MORE INFORMATION

See section 16.2.4 of the *American Medical Association Manual of Style* (AMA 1989).

PRINCIPLE 158. MASTER THE ELEMENTS OF A HIGH-QUALITY FIGURE.

Table 24–7 shows a checklist for creating a quality figure.

CHAPTER 25.

Discussion

FOCUSING THE DISCUSSION

PRINCIPLE 159. START THE DISCUSSION WITH YOUR MOST IMPORTANT POINT.

Your discussion should start with one sentence that clearly shows that your paper contains **new** information. Either accept or reject your original null hypothesis. If you are unsure how to start, you can always begin with: "We found that . . ."; then describe your primary findings and explain their importance. Never start with a dull history lesson!

PRINCIPLE 160. CONFINE THE DISCUSSION TO YOUR RESULTS AND COMPARISONS BETWEEN OTHER PUBLICATIONS AND YOUR RESULTS.

The Discussion is completely different from the Results. The Discussion is the place to discuss the **implications** of your findings, not simply repeat them. In the Discussion, do not discuss any findings that you did not present in the Results. **Confine the Discussion to the data that your study generated.**

ANTICIPATING PITFALLS IN THE DISCUSSION

PRINCIPLE 161. PROVIDE PRACTICAL INFORMATION.

In the Discussion, extract useful information from your data by interpreting the results and drawing conclusions. Most readers prefer pragmatic, "how-to" knowledge. To provide it, separate the science from the rhetoric. Also, remember that obvious leaps of logic will annoy editors.

PRINCIPLE 162. DISCIPLINE YOURSELF TO STICK TO YOUR SUBJECT AND KEEP THE DISCUSSION FOCUSED.

Do not go off on tangents. Good papers have a targeted Discussion. Many Discussion sections are too long and tend to recapitulate information given in the Results. Ask yourself: "Is all of the Discussion relevant?" Stay focused, and make a central point about one major topic.

PRINCIPLE 163. DESCRIBE THE NEW INFORMATION THAT YOUR PAPER PROVIDES.

Anticipate and avoid the most common reviewer criticism: **"This is nothing new!"**

(◎) VITAL POINT

Unoriginal, predictable, or trivial results guarantee rejection.

PRINCIPLE 164. COMPARE YOUR STUDY WITH PREVIOUS STUDIES.

Ask yourself: "What comparisons and contrasts do the experts in this field want to see?" Discuss how your results compare with landmark papers. Try to critique—concisely—the major studies most similar to yours.

When your conclusion differs dramatically from published reports, explain why. Do not dismiss earlier studies flippantly; those authors might be asked to review your manuscript. When you contradict published work, be honest, but be diplomatic.

◎ VITAL POINT

Say what you mean, mean what you say, but don't say it mean.

Write the Discussion as if you are talking with the reader. Imagine that the authors of the landmark papers on your subject are sitting around a table, listening as you discuss your findings and their publications. If necessary, explain how your measuring method differed from theirs. For example: Are the measurements parallel? Can you present your results in the same units of measurement to allow comparison? How were your methods an improvement over previous studies?

PRINCIPLE 165. OVERCOME REVIEWERS' INITIAL NEGATIVE REACTIONS.

Reviewers often start with the assumption that your paper does not add anything new. You can use subheadings to present your data in logical sections that anticipate the reviewer's response: **"This work has been done before."** This type of organization will help prove that it has not.

Remember that the peer review process has a "tendency to select against novel work" (Olson 1990). Because many reviewers strongly resist new ideas, novel or controversial findings need extra support.

Reviewers also may wonder about confounding factors that are not mentioned (e.g., nutritional status, social problems, the hospital's level of care). Anticipate the major concerns of reviewers and address them in the Discussion. If some of these factors could skew your data and affect your results, explain why you did not measure them. Moreover, from your experience, identify important variables for future study.

PRINCIPLE 166. OFFER ONLY SPECIFIC CRITICISM.

Making a sweeping critical statement is like throwing a boomerang, so be prepared.

PRINCIPLE 167. KEEP THE DISCUSSION SHORT.

Reviewers and editors report that the Discussion typically is too long and often flawed (see Figures 12–1 and 23–1). Do not force the reviewer to say:

 The Discussion should be shortened.

According to reviewers, wordiness is the most common writing problem (see Figure 32–1). Rewrite, using the fewest words possible. To produce crisp writing, **find and delete unnecessary words.** For example, many sentences begin with unnecessary words. Many sentences can be improved simply by deleting the words "a," "the," and "that."

If you have trouble deleting any of your hard work, save the deleted sections in another file. You may be able to use these sections for another paper, possibly a literature review.

DISCUSSING IMPLICATIONS

PRINCIPLE 168. DISCUSS THE INTERRELATION OF KEY VARIABLES.

Explain how the different measures of poor outcome are interrelated. Show how the cause and effect relations are biologically plausible. Describe whether the key variables are interrelated or independent. Explain whether screening tests could be used in combination to increase their predictive value.

Most statistical software packages can create a *correlation matrix,* which is a grid that shows the interrelation among variables. Although this matrix usually is much too detailed for publication, you should refer to it when you write the Discussion.

PRINCIPLE 169. EXPLAIN YOUR RATIONALE FOR RESEARCH JUDGMENTS.

Describe any unusual methods or analyses that you used, and explain why you deviated from the usual methods. For example, explain your motivation for deciding on the **sample size,** the definitions of outcome, and the statistical tests. Can you provide any support for these decisions?

PRINCIPLE 170. DISCUSS THE FINANCIAL IMPLICATIONS OF YOUR FINDINGS.

In the past, many medical research papers were written without any mention of money. Now, however, with the changes in health care financing, most reviewers expect to see some discussion of the financial ramifications (e.g., a cost–benefit analysis). If possible, compare and discuss the cost and duration of hospital stay, especially for the important subgroups. What are the costs of various types of treatment? How do your results relate to current issues in health care reform? How is this topic important at a time when health care dollars are shrinking? Explain the financial implications of the outcome and trends that you report. Discuss how your findings could be used by managed care administrators or patients who are trying to balance optimal care with cost control.

PRINCIPLE 171. SPECULATE INTELLIGENTLY.

State what is speculation. Avoid gross speculation. If you cannot provide evidence to support your opinion, expect a reviewer to tell you to delete the sentence. As one editor suggested: "Keep the Discussion lively, related to the results, but speculate with intelligence."

PRINCIPLE 172. CONSIDER ALTERNATIVE EXPLANATIONS FOR YOUR RESULTS.

In the Discussion, consider the opposing point of view by taking a devil's advocate position. Do not wait for a reviewer to play this role. **Identify the strengths and note the weaknesses of your study.** Most papers are improved by adding a few paragraphs under a subheading such as "Limitations of the Study." Address these questions: What problems occurred during your study? If you had to repeat the study and had unlimited money, what would you do differently? What are the weaknesses in your Methods? As experienced researchers know, you cannot believe all analysis at face value. Often, waiting for corroboration before acting on data is the best policy.

State whether your study was definitive or preliminary. Provide a biologically plausible explanation of how your findings could be associated with the outcome reported.

PRINCIPLE 173. BE SKEPTICAL OF PUBLISHED WORK.

One reviewer identified the following common mistake in analyzing data:

> Failure to consider the "null" hypothesis. Most clinicians assume that any published report is true and, after reading an article, unconsciously add their own name to the author list. This is especially true for younger doctors and students. It is safer to assume that the author is wrong, then see if he or she can overcome your skepticism.

Another reviewer said that a common problem occurs when people read only the conclusions, and not the body of the paper, or do not compare the results with published reports.

In your Introduction and Discussion, do not simply summarize published papers: critically evaluate their methodology, findings, and conclusions. For example: Are their conclusions based on recent data and a large sample size? Are the data drawn from a population that is appropriate for your needs?

DISCUSSING LIMITATIONS

PRINCIPLE 174. RECOGNIZE AND DISCUSS SELECTION BIAS.

Explain how the people who were selected for the study differ from those who were not selected. For example, during your chart review, were you missing more private patients than clinic patients? Do not misinterpret your results and present erroneous information. In the Methods, you should have stated which subjects were excluded and when they were excluded. In the Discussion, explain why you excluded patients with other severities of the study condition.

If your point has been proven for other populations, explain why the population that you studied is different and required to further prove the point.

Example 25–1.

People with depression might be particularly willing to respond to a questionnaire on depression, but then obviously, the results would suffer from selection bias.

PRINCIPLE 175. DISCUSS THE IMPLICATIONS OF ANALYZING ONLY RESPONDENTS.

For mailed questionnaires, explain how your sample of valid respondents differed from those who did not respond. For example, a problem would occur if 50% of the potential respondents were men and only 25% of the actual respondents were men. If you surveyed a local group, explain how your sample differed from subjects more broadly distributed across the country or even the world.

Anticipate questions from reviewers such as:

> If only 40% of subjects have these two conditions, why did you limit your study to these conditions? How would the other 60% be affected? How does your sample of 20 subjects differ from others with the same condition?

PRINCIPLE 176. DISCUSS PREDICTION CAUTIOUSLY.

For cross-sectional studies, explain that you understand that correlation does not equal causation. With this type of study design, avoid making strong conclusions regarding prediction and the development of conditions. Carefully interpret findings about risk factors that you assume antedated conditions.

PRINCIPLE 177. BE MODEST.

When you describe your study or a finding with the words "the first," "only," or "largest series," modesty requires that you add "known to us." Alternatively, you can write: "We are aware of no published reports that describe . . ." To convince the reader that your statement is true, explain how you conducted your literature search.

PRINCIPLE 178. DESCRIBE YOUR FINDINGS WITH APPROPRIATE BALANCE.

Use words such as **"proves"** cautiously; **"indicates"** usually is more appropriate. Also, phrases such as **"solves an important problem"** are too enthusiastic and therefore inappropriate. Do not overstate the importance of your findings. Show the evidence and discuss it, but remain understated and objective.

PRINCIPLE 179. DESCRIBE THE STRENGTHS AND LIMITATIONS OF YOUR FOLLOW-UP.

Reviewers often are interested in long-term follow-up data. For journals that require long-term follow-up, give the minimum and median follow-up times in the Results. Also, compare your follow-up with that of published studies. If reviewers think that the follow-up is too short, they may reject the paper. In the discussion of the paper's limitations, explain how your sample differs from the general population or the ideal sample. Reviewers may wonder whether the findings are skewed because your sample has a disproportionately high or low incidence of the risk factor.

PRINCIPLE 180. IDENTIFY A "CONTROL GROUP" IN THE LITERATURE.

If your study does not have an ideal control group, you may be able to use information from published studies to strengthen your Discussion. Although a control group from the literature is not a substitute for an actual control group, it is better than no comparison at all.

PRINCIPLE 181. DISCUSS ANY SURPRISING FINDINGS.

Point out any results that readers will find striking, even if the result was not intended or the variable was not important. For example, if the sensitivities are all less than 50%, you must elaborate on this situation. If you do not address unusual findings, reviewers will give your Discussion a poor rating.

PRINCIPLE 182. DISCUSS THE PROBLEMS ASSOCIATED WITH SMALL SAMPLE SIZE.

Tables often show large differences that are not statistically different. These differences might be caused by large variations in the measurements or by the inclusion of too few subjects. Discuss any limitations caused by a small sample size. If you did not find statistically significant differences because the sample size was small or the incidence was low, estimate the sample size at which these differences would appear significant. Also discuss the rationale for your sample size. Addressing these issues is far better than waiting for an editor to point them out in a rejection letter.

CONCLUSIONS

PRINCIPLE 183. CONCLUDE THE DISCUSSION WITH A "BOLT OF LIGHTNING."

The body of a good paper is a thunderbolt in reverse: it begins with thunder (the Introduction) and ends with lightning (the conclusions). Quality papers end with strong, clear conclusions.

Clearly state your recommendations so that reviewers do not say:

 What do the authors recommend?

 No recommendations are made as to what the clinician is to do with this information. It is interesting that differences in X exist, but how are we to alter management of these patients based on this?

Your summary statement, usually the final sentence in the Discussion, must capture what is important about your study. Do not end your Discussion with the weak statement that more research is needed. Remember that most people read the abstract, the conclusions, and then the Introduction—in that order.

PRINCIPLE 184. PROVIDE CAUTIOUS CONCLUSIONS THAT ARE FULLY SUPPORTED BY YOUR DATA.

Many writers give little attention to their conclusions. As a result, they often are the weakest link in a manuscript.

Unsupported conclusions are the most common and severe problem with interpretation (Figures 25–1 and 25–2). The conclusions must be drawn from the data presented in the manuscript. Any conclusions that are drawn from the statistical analysis must be justified in plain English, so polish your conclusion statement to avoid the following type of critique:

 The main weakness of this paper is that the authors neither consider nor control for many confounding factors. Therefore, the conclusion needs to be more conservative.

Answer the following questions: Are the conclusions correctly derived from the data presented? Can the conclusions be improved by narrowing the statement? Are the recommendations too general? Will the editor think that the conclusions are unwarranted?

Remember, even if your conclusions are correct, if they are not consistent with the evidence in your Results, your paper probably will be rejected.

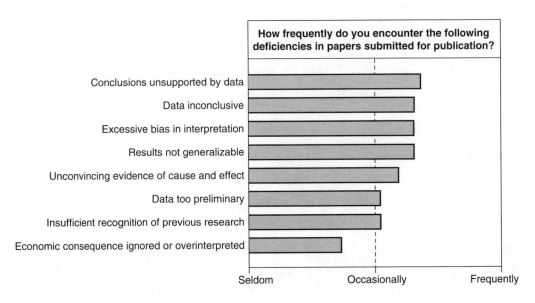

Figure 25–1. The frequency of interpretation problems. From question 8 of the Peer Review Questionnaire in Appendix B.

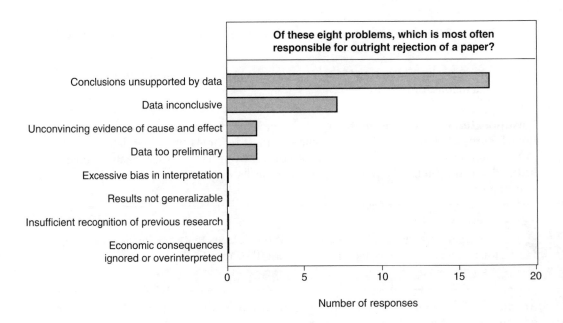

Figure 25–2. Interpretation problems and rejection. From question 9 of the Peer Review Questionnaire in Appendix B.

Anticipate reviewers saying that your conclusions:

- are inappropriate for the data.
- do not follow from the data.
- contradict the data and ignore important literature.

Many clinicians analyze their data incorrectly and then believe their interpretation.

PRINCIPLE 185. ANSWER THE QUESTION: "WHO CARES?"

What are the clinical implications of your findings? **If you do not discuss the clinical implications of your paper, it probably will be rejected.**

To avoid this problem, offer precise, concrete suggestions. Include data and references to show that your suggestions could improve outcome. Otherwise, reviewers may say:

> Why is this research question important? The Introduction and the Discussion need more details about the clinical applications of these findings.

Consider adding a section under the subheading **"Practical Considerations and Future Implications."** In this section, answer the following questions: Can you think of more interesting ways to look at your results? If you were a patient with the condition under study, how could these findings be useful? If you were the CEO of an HMO, how would these results be helpful? Of course, also explain how your study can help clinicians who treat patients with the condition under study.

PRINCIPLE 186. LIMIT CONCLUSIONS TO THE BOUNDARIES OF THE STUDY.

Conclusions drawn from uncontrolled retrospective data must be conservative. Will the reviewer think that your conclusions are sound based on the design of the study? For example, if no patients in your study died, reviewers might wonder how you can draw conclusions about morbidity and mortality. If your study was not a randomized clinical trial, interpret your findings carefully, especially those regarding treatment and outcome.

PRINCIPLE 187. DESCRIBE PRECISELY WHAT FURTHER RESEARCH IS NEEDED.

If you recommend additional research, explain why. For example, if you conclude that a larger sample is needed to permit more statistically significant conclusions, explain why your paper makes a contribution despite this problem. Otherwise, the reviewer might agree with you, send the manuscript back, and encourage you to enlarge your own sample.

CHAPTER 26.

References

CREATING A HIGH-QUALITY REFERENCE SECTION

PRINCIPLE 188. ALLOW ENOUGH TIME TO CREATE A FLAWLESS REFERENCE SECTION.

Many authors do not realize the importance that editors place on an accurate reference section. Present the reference section properly for the target journal. Use full-length articles from peer-reviewed journals. Papers that are submitted for publication, but not officially accepted, are not allowed as references by most journals. For many journals, abstracts are not allowed unless they are published in a journal. Refer to the target journal's guidelines.

A paper that is accepted for publication, but not yet published, may be cited as a reference. Add "in press" in parentheses in place of the volume and page numbers, and submit a copy of the paper with your manuscript. Update this reference before your paper is published.

When you are planning your study and writing early drafts, be sure that the reference citations are 100% correct the first time. Including sloppy or incomplete references, such as "Smith 1996," in these early drafts creates unnecessary work later.

An all-encompassing broad bibliography is viewed as a major flaw in a clinical research paper. Limit references to key citations, and avoid citing every publication on the subject. Look for appropriate, recent, or review references in journals with large circulations. Including 40 references usually is adequate for clinical research papers (Halsey 1994), but some journals limit the number to 20.

Double check your paper for statements that require references, especially statements that do not agree with the work of most investigators. Otherwise, reviewers may say:

 The bibliography does not cite many important papers.

PRINCIPLE 189. PLACE REFERENCE CITATIONS PROPERLY.

For most journals, place the citation number directly after the name of the cited author, not at the end of the sentence. When you report the work of several authors without naming them, however, place the citation number at the end of the sentence (e.g., "Previous reports have shown an incidence of 50%.[13,24,29]"). In the text, superscript the reference numbers or place them in parentheses or square brackets, depending on the journal's style.

REFERENCING SYSTEMS

PRINCIPLE 190. LEARN THE DIFFERENCES AMONG THE MAJOR REFERENCING SYSTEMS.

The three major systems are:

1. **Citation-Order, Citation-by-Reference, or Vancouver System:** References are numbered and listed in the order in which they are cited in the text. For medical journals, this system is the most common.

2. **Author–Date, Name-and-Year, or Harvard System:** References are cited in the text with the last name of the primary author and the year of publication. The reference list is arranged alphabetically by the authors' names. This system is also called the "APA" (American Psychological Association) system.
3. **Alphabet–Number System:** References are listed in alphabetical order according to the primary author's last name and cited by numbers in the text.

⊕ FOR MORE INFORMATION

The details of these systems vary from journal to journal, so as always follow the guidelines for the target journal. Refer to the *Publication Manual of the American Psychological Association* (APA 1994) for legal references or journals that follow the APA system.

Appendix A describes standard methods of referencing various sources. Researchers sometimes call these Uniform Requirements the "Vancouver style" (see Appendix A) because the Committee first met in Vancouver.

PRINCIPLE 191. FORMAT REFERENCES CORRECTLY FOR THE TARGET JOURNAL.

If you submit a paper with references that follow the format of another journal, the reviewers and editors may think that your paper was rejected by another journal. You probably will want to avoid this.

For references that are difficult to obtain, you can direct the reader to the source (e.g., "available from . . .").

⊕ FOR MORE INFORMATION

See the *List of Journals Indexed in Index Medicus* (see Appendix D) for the appropriate abbreviation for each journal. The list is published each year in the January issue of *Index Medicus*.

The *American Medical Association Manual of Style* lists the *Index Medicus* abbreviations for many common journals and is an excellent reference book to keep on your desk while you write a paper.

REFERENCING STATISTICAL SOFTWARE

The statistical software used in your study should have been described in the Methods as in the following examples.

Example 26–1.

All statistical analyses were performed with standard statistical software (SAS, Cary, NC; BMDP, Los Angeles, CA).

Analysis was conducted with the statistical programs Statview, Version 4.1 (Abacus, Concepts, Berkeley, CA), and Stata, Version 4 (Stata, College Station, TX).

In addition, providing a complete reference for the software manual is helpful as in the following examples.

Example 26–2.

1. SAS User's Guide. 4th ed. Vol. 1. Version 6. Cary, NC: SAS Institute; 1989.
2. Dixon WJ, editor. BMDP Statistical Software Manual. Berkeley (CA): University of California Press; 1992.
3. Norusis MJ. SPSS for Windows: advanced statistics. Release 6.0. Chicago: Statistical Package for the Social Sciences; 1993. p. 1–30.
4. Dean AG, Dean JA, Coulombier D, et al. Epi Info: a word processing, database, and statistics program for epidemiology on microcomputers. Version 6. Atlanta: Centers for Disease Control and Prevention; 1994.
5. Gustafson T. True Epistat Reference Manual. Version 5.0. Richardson (TX): Epistat Services; 1994.
6. Egret Reference Manual. Seattle: Statistics and Epidemiological Research Corporation; 1990.

POLISHING THE REFERENCES

PRINCIPLE 192. CHECK THE REFERENCES TO ENSURE THAT MINOR DETAILS ARE CORRECT.

Double check all references for accuracy of citation, attribution, format, and completeness. Also be sure that each reference is cited correctly in the text. If your time is limited, consider hiring someone to check that your references are 100% correct.

⊕ FOR MORE INFORMATION

See the American Medical Writers Association or International Medical Communications (see Appendix D) for freelance help.

Editors and copyeditors may return manuscripts that have even minor reference problems (e.g., incorrect punctuation, incorrect use of *Index Medicus* abbreviations).

Verify each reference with the photocopy of the paper (which you should have organized in a binder), and be sure that the cited references say what you think they say. Many errors are found in the reference section. Editors and reviewers cannot tell how carefully you conducted your research; therefore, many will look at the details of your references to assess the quality of your work.

PRINCIPLE 193. USE MODERN SOFTWARE PROGRAMS TO HELP ORGANIZE REFERENCES.

The software programs that organize and reformat your references have become quite sophisticated and can save time if you have many references or have to resubmit your paper to a journal with a different reference style.

⊕ FOR MORE INFORMATION

See End Note, ProCite, and Reference Manager (see Appendix D).

PRINCIPLE 194. REMEMBER TO CITE COAUTHORS.

When you name an author in your text, give the coauthors credit too. If you are discussing the work of one author, use "he" or "she"; if the study has two or more authors, use "they."

Example 26–3.

One author:

Lathers-McGillan[1] described Y. She reported that . . .

Two authors:

Jones and Wagner[2] reported X. They found that . . .

Three or more authors:

Smith et al.[3] found Z. They reported that . . .

The term "et al." means "and others." It is an abbreviation for two Latin terms: *et alii* (masculine) and *et aliae* (feminine). Journal style for citing multiple authors varies. Some use "et al.," which may or may not have a period and may or may not be italicized. Other journals avoid "et al." and alternate among the following (Halsey 1994):

- Smith and associates
- Smith and colleagues
- Smith and coworkers

CHAPTER 27.

Special Situations

ABSTRACTS FOR CONFERENCE COMPETITIONS

PRINCIPLE 195. SELECT HIGH-PROBABILITY CATEGORIES FOR CONFERENCES.

When you submit an abstract for a conference competition, remember that the likelihood of acceptance usually is higher for program categories that have the fewest submissions. If the abstract application form offers several valid choices, check the topic category that you anticipate will have the fewest submissions.

PRINCIPLE 196. CONSIDER THE "HOT" TOPICS FOR THE CONFERENCE.

Ask about the annual featured topics of the conference. The acceptance rate for these topics typically is high. Study last year's proceedings to determine the characteristics of accepted abstracts. For example, do they include tables in the abstract? You can use a literature search to show how your findings fill an important gap. Use contemporary terminology, and demonstrate the timeliness of your study.

PRINCIPLE 197. WRITE YOUR ABSTRACT WELL AHEAD OF THE DEADLINE, AND TAKE THE TIME TO REFINE IT.

Start working on your abstract at least 1 month before the submission deadline. Search the literature, meet with your coauthors several times to brainstorm, and submit your abstract for internal review. Then rewrite it based on the reactions of your colleagues.

ELECTRONIC PUBLISHING

PRINCIPLE 198. PREPARE FOR ELECTRONIC PUBLISHING.

If you do not have the skills or equipment to communicate by E-mail and access the Internet from your computer, make this investment soon. Although you may be skeptical about whether this effort will be worth your time and money, after you try it, you will be convinced.

Accessing the Internet can be frustrating at first, so you may want to ask a friend or a computer consultant to help you. You need a fast personal computer, a fast modem, and a fast Internet Service Provider (ISP). The latest version of Microsoft Windows will make this work easier. If your computer system seems slow when accessing information on the Internet, ask a computer consultant how to reconfigure your memory, files, and buffers.

When you have access to the Internet, you can explore the Web sites (http://www . . .) listed in Appendix D. Table 27–1 defines a few basic Internet terms that are helpful to know. A good place to begin is the National Library of Medicine. You can perform a free MEDLINE literature search at the following site: "http://www.ncbi.nlm.nih.gov/PubMed/.

Table 27–1.	Basic Internet Terms
Term	*Definition*
BBS	Bulletin Board System
FAQ	Frequently Asked Questions
FTP	File Transfer Protocol
html	Hypertext Markup Language
http	Hypertext Transfer Protocol
Internet	International Network of computers
ISP	Internet Service Provider
URL	Uniform Resource Locator, for example, http://www.wwilkins.com
Usernet	Global bulletin board
WAIS	Wide-Area Information Servers
www	World Wide Web

⊕ FOR MORE INFORMATION

For information on purchasing a personal computer, you may want to consult Compaq (see Appendix D).

P
O
W
E
R

EDITING

Key Questions to Answer in the Editing Phase:

- *Have you said what you intended to say?*

- *Are you asking too much of the reader?*

CHAPTER 28.

Preparing Your Manuscript for Submission

SEEKING INTERNAL PEER REVIEW

PRINCIPLE 199. HAVE YOUR MANUSCRIPT PEER REVIEWED INTERNALLY.

Let us assume that you have finished the Planning, Observing, and Writing phases. At this point, many unsuccessful medical writers submit their manuscripts for publication and POW! They are rejected. Successful writers find the patience and determination to complete the remaining two phases of the POWER principles: Editing and Revising. As the writer, Silvana Clark (1994) said: "There's so little traffic on the extra mile."

 VITAL POINT

Before you submit your paper to a journal, ask several colleagues to review it, especially those who are experienced in journal publishing.

Try to find unbiased colleagues who can provide stringent reviews. Give a double-spaced copy of the manuscript, for comments, and a copy of the internal peer review form (Figure 28–1) to each coauthor, several colleagues, and your biostatistician and ask for a critical review.

Ironically, many people are offended by how they are thanked in the acknowledgments. For this reason, give a copy of the acknowledgments to everyone you thank (to be sure that they are happy with the way you characterize them, their job title, and their contribution to the paper). Obtaining written permission from all persons named in the acknowledgments is a wise step—even if it is not required by the target journal.

When you ask colleagues to review your manuscript, indicate where you are planning to submit your paper and ask your colleagues to do the following:

1. Mark any sections that are difficult to understand.
2. Summarize their reactions to the paper in the margins.
3. Mark where they stopped reading and any sections that they skipped.

Address your colleagues' concerns and also edit your paper to avoid the following types of comments:

 I found the manuscript somewhat difficult to follow in places.

 I am uncertain as to how you arrived at the numbers X, Y, and Z in the Results. They do not correspond to the tables. I am confused. Please explain.

Figure 28–1. Internal peer review form.

The purpose of this form is to help medical researchers to critique

their colleagues' manuscripts before submission.

General instructions:

With a red pen, mark the sections that require clarification.

Highlight areas in which the wording or numbers are confusing or incorrect.

Describe the three major weaknesses of this paper:

I.

II.

III.

Check any of the following areas that are weak and require additional work before submission:

_____ Importance and originality of the subject for the target journal

_____ Adequacy of the study design/appropriateness of the approach

_____ Adequacy of the patients or materials studied

_____ Accuracy of the interpretation of the results

_____ Statistical analysis

_____ Relevance of the Discussion section

_____ Soundness of the conclusions

_____ Appropriateness of the references

_____ Appropriateness, clarity, and adequacy of the tables/figures

_____ Clarity of the presentation

_____ Accurateness and adequacy of the abstract

What additional information would you need to reproduce this study?

How would you strengthen the Discussion and analysis?

(Circle all that apply).

Which sections are too long?   Abstract Introduction Methods Results Discussion

Which sections are too short?   Abstract Introduction Methods Results Discussion

Which tables would you delete?   1   2   3   4   5   6   7   8+

Which figures would you delete?   1   2   3   4   5   6   7   8+

What conclusions would you draw from these results?

Which sections of this manuscript could be misunderstood?

What flaws are evident in the execution of this study?

How could the title be improved?

	No	Yes
Did this study raise and resolve an important question?	____	____
Does this manuscript follow the target journal's standard format?	____	____
Is the writing clear and concise?	____	____
Are the paragraphs organized to allow for intelligent skimming?	____	____
Are the units of measure included and abbreviated consistently?	____	____
Is this sudy interesting?	____	____

Figure 28–1. Internal peer review form   (continued).

Explain any apparent discrepancies between the text and the tables. Reread the Results, and delete any information that appears in the tables.

Do not rush to submit your paper. Remember, journals often spend months reviewing manuscripts. To increase the chance that your paper will be accepted, spend more time editing your writing to avoid the problems listed in Figures 28–2 and 28–3. Consider having your manuscript professionally edited, especially if your first language is not English.

⊕ FOR MORE INFORMATION

See the American Medical Writers Association or International Medical Communications in Appendix D for writing or editing assistance.

As you may remember from Figure 12–1, a priority during editing is to make each section the correct length.

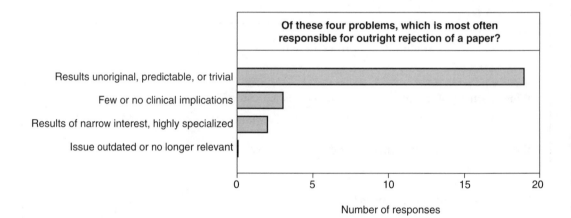

Figure 28–2. Topic problems that are responsible for rejection. From question 11 of the Peer Review Questionnaire in Appendix B.

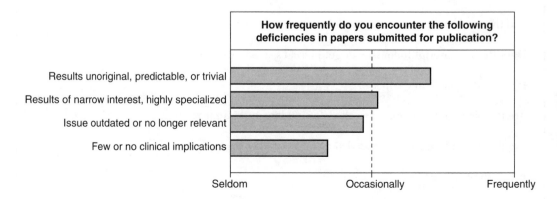

Figure 28–3. Frequency of topic problems. From question 10 of the Peer Review Questionnaire in Appendix B.

◎ VITAL POINT

A good rule is: Shorten the Introduction and Discussion; lengthen the Methods and Results.

PRINCIPLE 200. ASK A FRIEND OR COLLEAGUE OUTSIDE YOUR SPECIALTY TO CRITIQUE YOUR PAPER BEFORE YOU SUBMIT IT TO A JOURNAL WITH A GENERAL AUDIENCE.

Your manuscript may be too specialized or complicated for many readers. To anyone other than you and your coauthors, your writing may be impossible to understand.

Half of the manuscripts submitted to the *British Medical Journal* are quickly rejected for one of three reasons:

1. Lack of originality
2. Serious scientific flaws
3. Lack of importance to a general medical audience

Consider these points, and rewrite any sections that people outside your field may not understand. Although, at this point in the process some flaws cannot be eliminated, you must edit your paper until your message is clear and direct.

⊕ FOR MORE INFORMATION

If you plan to submit your article to a nursing journal, you may find the following books useful: Barnum (1995), Polit-O'Hara and Hungler (1995), and Sheridan and Dowdney (1986).

EDITING FOR BREVITY AND CLARITY

PRINCIPLE 201. ELIMINATE ALL JARGON.

Jargon is obscure, often pretentious, language with long or unnecessary words. Jargon in medical research papers causes countless problems and should be avoided. Within each specialty, medical researchers use distinctive words or phrases. The trouble occurs when authors must communicate with those outside their specialty, geographic area, or generation. The specialized terms then become gibberish.

When you must use a phrase that could be considered jargon, enclose the term in quotation marks and define it. After the initial explanation, do not repeat the quotation marks. Also avoid colloquialisms, clichés, and euphemisms (Table 28–1).

When you are editing, ask yourself: "Can I express my idea in a shorter, more direct, or less technical way?" Careful editing can change writing from turgid, bombastic, and pompous to plain English. Poor English is a common criticism and highly annoying to reviewers, so aim for clear, jargon-free writing.

As Martin Fischer (Daintith 1989) said: "You must learn to talk clearly. The jargon of scientific terminology which rolls off your tongues is mental garbage."

Table 28–1.   Examples of Colloquialisms, Clichés, Euphemisms, and Slang

Colloquialisms and clichés

- The common thread
- Landed a patient in the ICU
- State of the art
- Kept in mind
- On top of this
- By a wide margin
- By a clear margin
- Big DRG losers

Euphemisms

- Nonsurvivors
- The rat was sacrificed

Slang

- Lab
- Prepped
- Temp

PRINCIPLE 202. USE SIMPLE DECLARATIVE SENTENCES.

Try to reword sentences that begin with the phrases shown in Table 28–2. This rewording should make your writing more professional. Some words and phrases are overused as sentence beginnings. Table 28–3 lists suggestions for simplifying or improving sentences.

Sometimes two sentences are closely related, but cannot be combined. In this situation, you may be able to edit the first few words of the second sentence to provide a transition from the first sentence. Table 28–4 shows some examples of transitional phrases.

Avoid starting a sentence with a number. Even if the number is written out, the sentence probably will be awkward.

Example 28–1.

"One hundred ninety-seven . . ." is a bad way to start any sentence.

PRINCIPLE 203. ELIMINATE SUPERFLUOUS COMMAS AND DASHES.

Do not insert a comma every time the reader needs to inhale. **Most manuscripts can be improved by deleting several commas;** however, commas are often needed after a beginning transitional word or phrase (e.g., "Conversely," "In fact,").

Table 28–2. Sentence Beginnings to Avoid

As a matter of fact
Based on the fact that (change to "Because")
Due to (try "Because")
Here
Hopefully
In a very real sense
In light of the fact that (try "Because")
In order to (try "To")
In other words
In the event that (change to "If")
It goes without saying
It has been reported by Smith that (change to "Smith reported that")
It has been shown
It is important to note that
It may be
It was found that
More importantly (change to "More important")
Note well that
Of course
Out of this study population
Past and present research has outlined
That is to say
There (change to an active statement)
They
Whether it be
Yet

Table 28–3. Sentence Beginnings to Use Sparingly

However (move it to the middle of the sentence)
In addition
In general (try "Overall")
It (replace with the phrase that "it" stands for)
Therefore (move it to the middle of the sentence)

Table 28–4. Transitional Phrases
Although
From this number
For these reasons
Further
In contrast
Moreover
Similarly
These included
This decrease suggests
This relationship can be
Thus

Insert a comma before "and" in a series of three or more items, such as A, B, C, and D. The same rule applies to "or."

Use semicolons, not commas, to separate numbered items in a series. For example:

The inclusion criteria were as follows: (1) ____; (2) ____; and (3) ____.

In medical writing, a comma usually is preferred in place of a dash. Save the dash for setting off words that require special emphasis.

⊕ FOR MORE INFORMATION

The Gregg Reference Manual by William A. Sabin (1992) is an excellent writing reference book that is both well organized and easy to understand.

PRINCIPLE 204. RECOGNIZE WHEN TO USE "THAT" AND "WHICH."

Restrictive clauses are phrases that do not limit the reference of a modified word or phrase. They do not require commas and usually are preceded by "that" rather than "which." Restrictive clauses are essential to the meaning of the sentence. For example: The antibiotic that was most effective was ampicillin. In this sentence, "that" introduces an essential clause. Without the clause, the meaning of the sentence is changed: The antibiotic was ampicillin.

Nonrestrictive (descriptive) clauses are phrases that are set off by commas. They usually are preceded by "which." Nonrestrictive clauses are not essential to the meaning of the sentence; they provide additional information. For example: Ampicillin, which was used in Group II, was most effective. In this sentence, "which" introduces a nonessential clause. Without the clause, the basic meaning of the sentence is not changed: Ampicillin was most effective.

Compare the meaning of the following sentences:

1. Surgery is required for Stage II tumors, which do not respond to chemotherapy.
2. Surgery is required for Stage II tumors that do not respond to chemotherapy.

PRINCIPLE 205. USE PROFESSIONAL SYMBOLS.

You can use Greek letters, foreign accents, and mathematical and other symbols in your manuscript, even if they are not displayed on your personal computer keyboard. These symbols can make your paper look more professional (e.g., $\pm$ rather than +/−). To use these symbols on most personal computers, follow these steps:

1. Hold down the alternate (Alt) key.
2. Type the corresponding three-digit (ASCII) code on the numeric keypad.
3. Release the Alt key.

Table 28–5 shows symbols that you can use in your manuscripts.

PRINCIPLE 206. USE THE WORD "DATA" AS YOU WOULD USE THE WORD "NUMBERS."

The following point is minor, but a favorite of many statistical reviewers: "Data" is the plural form of the rarely used word "datum."

Table 28–5. Additional Symbols and Codes

Symbol	Three-Digit Code Alt+	Symbol	Three-Digit Code Alt+	Symbol	Three-Digit Code Alt+
⌂	127	Ü	154	Σ	228
Ç	128	¢	155	σ	229
ü	129	£	156	μ	230
é	130	¥	157	τ	231
â	131	₨	158	Φ	232
ä	132	ƒ	159	Θ	233
à	133	á	160	Ω	234
å	134	í	161	δ	235
ç	135	ó	162	∞	236
ê	136	ú	163	ø	237
ë	137	ñ	164	ε	238
è	138	Ñ	165	∩	239
ï	139	ª	166	≡	240
î	140	º	167	±	241
ì	141	¿	168	≥	242
Ä	142	⌐	169	≤	243
Å	143	¬	170	⌠	244
É	144	½	171	⌡	245
æ	145	¼	172	÷	246
Æ	146	¡	173	≈	247
ô	147	«	174	°	248
ö	148	»	175	•	249
ò	149	▓	176	·	250
û	150	α	224	√	251
ù	151	β	225	ⁿ	252
ÿ	152	Γ	226	²	253
Ö	153	π	227	■	254

Table 28–6. How to Use the Word "Data"	
Problematic Usage	*Preferred Usage*
This data	These data
Less data	Fewer data
Much data	Many data
Data was	Data were

To determine whether your sentence is correct, replace the word "**data**" with the word "**numbers**."

In some cases, you can substitute another word to avoid awkwardness. For example:

A sentence that begins "Little data is available . . ." can be rewritten as "Little information is available . . . ."

Table 28–6 shows how to use the word "data."

PRINCIPLE 207. SUBMIT A PROFESSIONAL-LOOKING MANUSCRIPT.

Most journals prefer that authors avoid using boldface, italics, or underlining. If you want to italicize a word, underline it in your manuscript. Also avoid using quotation marks unless you are quoting someone directly or using a word or phrase in an unusual sense (e.g., Preoperative "fine-tuning" consisted of . . .).

Never submit a single-spaced manuscript. Most journal editors prefer double-spaced papers, and a few (including the *New England Journal of Medicine*) request triple-spaced copy.

Do not right-justify the text, and do not break words at the end of a line. Print the final version on a laser printer, not a dot-matrix or ink-jet printer. Use a type size of at least 10 points.

Be sure that you are submitting a complete package. Double check that each copy has an abstract and includes the correct number of tables and figures. Finally, verify that the final manuscript meets all of the requirements listed in the guidelines for authors.

CHAPTER 29.

Small, but Significant
Points to Consider

PRINCIPLE 208. FOLLOW THE TARGET JOURNAL'S STYLE.

Each journal has its own style. Check the target journal's format for style points (e.g., whether to use "percent" or "%"). For most journals, numbers less than ten are written out, unless they appear with percentages or units of time or measure. Within each sentence, however, be consistent, regardless of whether a number is less than ten.

Example 29–1.

Group I had a mean score of 25, and Group II had a mean score of 7 (not "seven").

Be alert to stylistic differences among journals. For example, uppercase (capital) P is preferred for *P* values in most journals, but not all. Before you submit your paper, check the relevant style points. These points may seem trival but journals want papers written in their style.

⊕ FOR MORE INFORMATION

Check a recent issue of the target journal, and refer to *The Gregg Reference Manual* (Sabin 1992) for specific style points.

Table 29–1 shows differences in house style among journals. Some of the style points suggested in this book are not followed by all journals.

You may think that because these points are minor, they are not important. However, you can increase the likelihood of acceptance if your paper looks as if it belongs in the target journal. More important, you can avoid errors that might occur if you leave too many changes for the copy editor.

Example 29–2.

A paper was published in which the outcome was defined in the manuscript as $\leq X$; however, the copy editor changed it to "greater than or equal to X."

Some journals do not allow text written in the first person. For these journals, make the types of changes shown in Table 29–2 before you submit your paper.

PRINCIPLE 209. USE SPACING THAT IS APPROPRIATE FOR THE PUNCTUATION.

Today, most authors prepare their own manuscripts on personal computers. Many never learned the fine points of typing, such as the convention of leaving two spaces after each period. Some word processing programs automatically prevent this problem so that the sentences look professional when justified, however, remember that most journal editors prefer manuscripts that are not right justified. Also, remember to include two spaces after a colon, but one space after a semicolon. Although these points may seem trivial, if you ignore them, your manuscript may look less than professional.

Table 29–1.   Examples of House Style Differences Among Journals

%	percent
$P < 0.001$	$p < 0.001$
less than 3.9	< 3.9
orthopaedic	orthopedic
Chi-square	chi-square
Figure	Fig
vs.	versus, v
Grams	g
follow-up	followup
in-hospital	inhospital
6-year	6-yr
Table 3	Table III
5	five
et al.	et al
one hundred ninety-seven	one-hundred-ninety-seven

Table 29–2.   Rephrasing From the First Person to the Third Person

First Person	*Third Person*
Our objective	The authors' objective
Our results	The current study
We analyzed	The authors analyzed
We are indebted to, We thank	The authors thank

PRINCIPLE 210. CREATE A PROFESSIONAL-LOOKING TITLE PAGE.

Appendix A indicates the general information that should be included on the title page but title pages are very journal-specific. The following are a few additional points:

- List only coauthors who meet the full criteria for authorship.
- Include each author's highest academic degree.
- Provide each author's current job title and institutional affiliation at the time the study was performed.
- Include the details of where and when the paper was presented.
- Use the two-letter postal abbreviation for your state (within the United States).
- Capitalize the first letter of each key word in the running title.
- Provide the full name (not just an acronym) of any funding agency for your project, and include the grant number.
- Every time that you edit or print your paper, put the current date on the title page so that you can verify that you are using the current version.

◎ VITAL POINT

Your goal is to make the editor think: "We can publish this paper without an inordinate amount of work."

CHAPTER 30.

Improving Your Writing

LEARNING FROM THE EXPERTS

PRINCIPLE 211. STUDY GEORGE ORWELL'S RULES.

George Orwell (1954) provided the following six rules for writing:

1. Never use a metaphor, simile, or other figure of speech which you are used to seeing in print.
2. Never use a long word where a short one will do.
3. If it is possible to cut a word out, always cut out.
4. Never use the passive where you can use the active.
5. Never use a foreign phrase, a scientific word, or a jargon word if you can think of an everyday English equivalent.
6. Break any of these rules sooner than say anything outright barbarous.

Many medical researchers ask about the use of the passive versus the active voice. In most cases, medical writing is improved by the use of the active voice, as Orwell advised. In some sentences, however, especially in the Methods section, the passive voice is preferred because it emphasizes what was performed rather than who performed it.

PRINCIPLE 212. APPLY THE GUIDELINES THAT ERNEST HEMINGWAY FOLLOWED.

Hemingway said that the following guidelines were "the best rules I ever learned in the business of writing":

1. Use short sentences.
2. Use short first paragraphs.
3. Use vigorous English.
4. Be positive, not negative.

PRINCIPLE 213. TAKE THOREAU'S ADVICE.

"Simplify, simplify, simplify," advised Thoreau. This advice certainly would improve most medical manuscripts, although it is ironic that Thoreau didn't follow his own advice and write: "Simplify."

PRINCIPLE 214. HEED THE ADVICE OF MEDICAL JOURNAL EDITORS.

Table 30–1 provides advice from editors.

PRINCIPLE 215. READ (OR REREAD) *THE ELEMENTS OF STYLE.*

You have heard this advice before, but it is worth repeating. No matter how experienced a writer you are, rereading this classic book by William Strunk, Jr., and E. B. White (1979) is worth your time.

Table 30–1.　Advice From Editors*
• Read and follow the instructions for authors.
• Read the journal and understand what our readers want, who they are, and the focus of the journal.
• Assure the clinical relevance and validity of the study.
• Think it out before.
• Present findings in perspective.
• Select only essential information to include.
• Put in all the information needed to make your case.
• Write it clearly.
• Be original and concise.
• Ask a respected neutral party to review your paper prior to submission.
• Have your paper professionally edited for English grammar.
• Shorten by one-fourth.
*From question 31 of the Peer Review Questionnaire in Appendix B.

PRINCIPLE 216. READ STYLE: TOWARD CLARITY AND GRACE.

This book by Joseph M. Williams (1995) is a readable, informative guide to grammar and writing. Williams provides details and examples to help authors follow vague guidelines such as: "Omit needless words" and "Be concise."

EDITING YOUR PAPER
FOR A MEDICAL JOURNAL

PRINCIPLE 217. INCLUDE INTERESTING EXAMPLES.

Whenever appropriate, provide interesting anecdotes to SHOW readers, rather than TELL them. In a medical manuscript, examples are appropriate if they are handled professionally.

PRINCIPLE 218. EDIT, EDIT, EDIT! CUT, CUT, CUT!

Although the importance of editing has been mentioned before Table 30–2 shows specific words and phrases that often can be cut to make your paper more professional.

PRINCIPLE 219. FIND AND REMOVE PROBLEM WORDS AND PHRASES.

Use your word processor to find the word "there." Delete it. Rewrite the sentence with an active verb (Payne 1965). Make sure that the reader understands who did what. These steps improve most sentences. See Table 30–3 for examples of sentences that are improved by deleting the word "there."

If you are submitting your paper to an American-based, English language publication, you often can improve your writing by following the suggestions shown in Tables 30–4 through 30–15.

Table 30–2.   Words and Phrases to Delete

and/or	fashion	rather (adjective)
as to	he/she	seem
best	individual	so that
case	majority	that have been
certainly	manner	that was
considerable	nature	that were
e.g.	needless to say	very
etc.	quite	

Table 30–3.   Examples of How Sentences Can Be Improved by Deleting the Word "There"

Original:	There has been an increase in the number of patients . . .
Improved:	More patients are . . .
Original:	There were no pulmonary emboli or deep wound infections.
Improved:	No pulmonary emboli or deep wound infections occurred.
Original:	There were 63 patients with . . .
Improved:	Sixty-three patients had . . .
Original:	Because there can be . . .
Improved:	Because X can exist . . .
Original:	There were seven pregnancies . . .
Improved:	Seven infants had . . .
Original:	There was a significant increase in adverse outcome . . .
Improved:	Adverse outcome increased significantly . . .
Original:	There is evidence to suggest that those who cease smoking . . .
Improved:	Those who cease smoking may . . .

Table 30–4.   Usage Problems

Problematic Usage	Preferred Usage
While most studies, where as most studies	whereas most studies
whilst 20.2% of those	whereas 20.2% of those
Since this was	Because this was
In this country	In the United States
Half the patients	One-half of the patients
reproducible methodology	reproducible method
analysis was done	analysis was performed
There are several limitations	This study has several limitations
over a short period	for a short period
similar to those above	similar to those used earlier
the above-listed criteria	the previously listed criteria
mentioned above	mentioned previously
prior to	before
parameter	characteristic
a HMO physician	an HMO physician
a SCI patient	a patient with SCI
the albumin was	the albumin concentration was
5-minute Apgar score <7	5 min Apgar score of less than 7
delivered before 37 weeks	delivered before 37 weeks of gestation
White's classification	the White classification
Out of 55 patients	Among the 55 patients
amongst cancer patients	among patients with cancer
Center for Disease Control	Centers for Disease Control and Prevention
mucus membrane	mucus (noun), mucous (adjective) membrane
data was utilized	data were used
investigator, who was blinded to	investigator, blinded to
This demonstrates	This shows
Data were collected on	Data were collected concerning
have good outcome	experience a good outcome
came to the identical conclusion	agreed
All chart data	All data from the charts
data established before	data collected before
a group of M.D.'s	a group of M.D.s
seven Ph.D.'s	seven Ph.D.s
Table 1 compares the risk factors.°	A comparison of the risk factors is shown in Table 1.

°Tables and Figures cannot compare.

Table 30–5. Describing Results From the Literature

Problematic Usage	Preferred Usage
has been shown to be	is
was found to be	was
In the X report, it was found that	The X report showed that
Smith et al looked at	Smith et al examined
One of the few studies on X is a paper by Smith et al.	Smith et al conducted one of the few studies on X.
The current study confirms previous results that indicate	The results of the current study agree with those from previous studies that indicated
X has been well studied showing	X has been studied extensively. Results have shown that
associated with:	associated with the following:
This finding is in contrast to reports for	This finding differs from those reported regarding
There have been studies comparing	Previous studies have compared
The literature reports	Several reports in the literature describe
It would appear that	It appears that

Table 30–6. Diction Problems

Problematic Usage	Preferred Usage
best	optimal, ideal
This method came about	This method was developed
due to	attributable to
get	(use a more specific verb, such as "become infected with")
gives	provides
The percent with X goes up	The percentage with X increased
just	(delete)
like	analogous to, similar to, such as
rest	remainder
show (sometimes a problem)	display, explain
We felt	We believe
They felt that	They believe that
works	functions
talk	describe, discuss

Table 30–7.   Capitalization Problems

Problematic Usage	Preferred Usage
Chi-Square	Chi-square, chi-square
class IV	Class IV
demerol	Demerol
fishers exact test	Fisher's exact test
Follow-Up	Follow-up (in a title)
Level 1 Trauma Center	level I trauma center
medicare and medicaid	Medicare and Medicaid
pearson product-moment correlation coefficient	Pearson product-moment correlation coefficient
pearson correlation coefficient	Pearson correlation coefficient
social security number	Social Security number
students t test	Student's t-test

Table 30–8.   Phrases to Transpose

Problematic Usage	Preferred Usage
with what is traditionally	with what traditionally is
independently able to walk	able to walk independently
has also been	also has been
as the source of data	as the data source
outcome has usually been	outcome usually has been
prospectively measure	measure prospectively
should also be examined	also should be examined
disease onset	onset of disease
patient characteristics	characteristics of the patients

Table 30–9.   British Diphthongs

Problematic Usage	Preferred Usage
labour	labor
haematocrit	hematocrit
haematology	hematology
orthopedic	orthopaedic
°Thrombocytopaenia	thrombocytopenia

°Misspelled as a diphthong.

Table 30–10.   Problems With Numbers

Problematic Usage	Preferred Usage
with an average of 5.2 years	(average, 5.2 years)
(range 28–92).	(range, 28–92 days).
(44/87)	(44 of 87)
The median score was 29.0.	The median score was 29 points.
Using an estimate of $1,000 per day	With an estimate of $1000 per patient per day of hospitalization
3 million a year	3 million per year
7 days	a stay of 7 days
beyond that limit	longer than the 7-day limit
stay beyond 11 days	stay in the hospital for longer than 11 days
one percent	1 percent, 1%
an albumin <3.4	an albumin concentration of <3.4
(Tables 2–4).	(Tables 2 to 4).
Patients were between 18–65 years of age.	Patients were between 18 and 65 years of age.
Of the 155, 79 patients had	Among the 155 patients, 79 had
There were over 70 million injuries.	More than 70 million injuries occurred.
1,600,000,000 dollars	$1.6 billion*
fall	decline, decrease
above	greater than
lower	lesser
level	concentration
rise	increase
below	less than
higher	greater
very few	only two patients
quite a small percentage	4%
practically all	98%

*One billion in the American system is 1,000,000,000 (10^9); however, in the British system, one billion is 1,000,000,000,000 (10^{12}). Be sure that the reader understands which system you are using.

Table 30–11. Hyphenated Terms

Problematic Usage	Preferred Usage
β Blockers	β-blockers
Cox proportional hazards model	Cox proportional-hazards model
diagnosis related group	diagnosis-related group
do not resuscitate orders	do-not-resuscitate orders
double blind study	double-blind study
double check	double-check (verb)
end expiratory pressure	end-expiratory pressure
end stage renal disease	end-stage renal disease
finetuning	fine-tuning
fluid containing cysts	fluid-containing cysts
follow up	follow-up (noun or adjective)
halflife	half-life
health care costs	health-care costs
high risk group	high-risk group
in depth study	in-depth study
intraabdominal surgery	intra-abdominal surgery
intraobserver	intra-observer
lactose containing food	lactose-containing food
little known study	little-known study
long term care	long-term care
metaanalysis	meta-analysis
needlestick	needle-stick
noninsulin dependent diabetes mellitus	non–insulin-dependent diabetes mellitus
over a two year period	during a 2-year period
part time employee	part-time employee
S/D ratio	S/D or S-D ratio
short term	short-term
six month review	6-month review
small bowel resection	small-bowel resection
small cell carcinoma	small-cell carcinoma
spinal cord disabled person	spinal cord–disabled person
spinal cord injured patients	spinal cord–injured patients
triple blinded	triple-blinded
third trimester values	third-trimester values
two sided t test	two-sided t-test
one tailed t test	one-tailed t-test
up to date report	up-to-date report
well established efficacy	well-established efficacy
Xray	X-ray (adjective or verb), X ray (noun)
The X ray indicated	The radiograph showed
An X ray was made	A radiograph was made
A X ray reading	An X-ray reading
a 8 hour procedure	an 8-hour procedure
a 80 year old patient	an 80-year-old patient
a 25 fold increase	a 25-fold increase

Table 30–12.   Prefixes and Numbers That Generally Require a Hyphen

Prefixes

- all-
- cross-
- ex-
- high-
- low-
- quasi-
- self-

Numbers

- twenty-one through ninety-nine

Fractions

- one-half
- two-thirds
- six-tenths

Table 30–13.   Terms That Do Not Require a Hyphen

Problematic Usage	*Preferred Usage*
African-American respondents	African American respondents
At base-line, X was 10.	At baseline, X was 10.
case-mix	case mix
check-list	checklist
co-author	coauthor
double-check	double check (noun)
fault-finding	faultfinding
follow-up	follow up (verb)
germ-free	germ free
died in-hospital	died in the hospital
health-care reform	health care reform
high-risk for pneumonia	high risk for pneumonia
inter-observer	interobserver
life-saving therapies	lifesaving therapies
multi-center	multicenter
non-compliant	noncompliant
non-fatal	nonfatal
non-operative	nonoperative
non-orthopaedic	nonorthopaedic

(continued)

Table 30–13. Terms That Do Not Require a Hyphen (*continued*)

Problematic Usage	Preferred Usage
non-parametric	nonparametric
non-smoker	nonsmoker
non-white	nonwhite
post-operative	postoperative
pre-existing	preexisting
proof-read	proofread
seat-belt	seat belt
set-up	set up (verb) setup (noun)
state-wide	statewide
step-wise	stepwise
straight-forward	straightforward
a ten-fold increase	a tenfold increase
vaccinations were up-to-date	vaccinations were up to date

Table 30–14. Words for Which the English Plural Is Preferred

Singular Form	Plural Form
amoeba	amoebas (not amoebae)
analysis	analyses
apparatus	apparatuses
appendix	appendixes (relating to a book), appendices (relating to anatomy)
cannula	cannulas
cranium	craniums
crisis	crises
focus	focuses
formula	formulas
hypothesis	hypotheses
index	indices (relating to mathematics), indexes (relating to a book)
matrix	matrices (relating to mathematics or medicine), matrixes (relating to other subjects)
myoma	myomas
schema	schemas
vortex	vortexes

Table 30–15.   Words for Which the Non-English Plural Is Preferred

Singular Form	Plural Form
alumna, alumnus	alumni
bacterium	bacteria
criterion	criteria
datum (rarely used)	data
decubitus	decubitus
erratum	errata
medium	media
minutia	minutiae
nucleus	nuclei
ovum	ova
phenomenon	phenomena
radius	radii
stigma	stigmata
stimulus	stimuli
stratum	strata

⊕ FOR MORE INFORMATION

If you have questions about hyphenation, remember to hyphenate anything that could be misread. Consult a comprehensive dictionary, such as the *American Heritage Dictionary* (1996) or *Merriam-Webster's Collegiate Dictionary* (1993) for guidelines on hyphenation. For medical words, see section 6.12 of the *American Medical Association Manual of Style* (AMA 1989). For general rules, *The Gregg Reference Manual* (Sabin 1992) and Table 6.1 of the *Chicago Manual of Style* (1993) are helpful.

CHAPTER 31.

Problematic Terms

PRINCIPLE 220. LEARN THE PROPER USE OF PROBLEMATIC WORD PAIRS.

Table 31–1 shows pairs of words that cause problems for many medical writers.

Avoid using "while" unless you mean "at the same time." "Compared with" usually is preferred to "compared to" for analysis of differences or similarities (Sabin 1992). **"Disinterested"** means "unbiased, impartial, or fair," whereas **"uninterested"** means "not interested in, bored, indifferent, or unconcerned."

⊕ FOR MORE INFORMATION

See Chapter 9 of the *American Medical Association Manual of Style* (AMA 1989) or a comprehensive dictionary, such as the *American Heritage Dictionary* (1996) or *Merriam-Webster's Collegiate Dictionary* (1993).

PRINCIPLE 221. USE FEW ABBREVIATIONS OR, BETTER YET, NONE.

Before you print a new draft of your paper, use your electronic spelling checker. However, do not use the automatic search and replace feature. Also consider using an electronic medical dictionary, such as *Stedman's Medical Dictionary* (see Appendix D). These tools can help you determine whether you are using too many abbreviations. Most abbreviations and acronyms within the text, tables, and figures should be deleted and the full term given. Limit abbreviations to chemical compounds and standard units of measure. Do not invent new abbreviations, such as those used for variable names in your statistical software package (e.g., GESTAGE). If you must use abbreviations, define each one the first time it is used.

◎ VITAL POINT

Papers that contain too many abbreviations are difficult to read, and papers that are difficult to read usually are rejected.

Many journals provide a list of approved abbreviations. Even these abbreviations must be used consistently. If you use a term only once or twice in your paper, do not abbreviate it.

Example 31–1.

The New England Journal of Medicine allows the following abbreviations: AIDS, ANOVA, ELISA, HDL, HIV, and NIDDM. It does not allow BUN, CNS, CSF, EKG, MI, qid, or RBC.

PRINCIPLE 222. BUY AND USE GRAMMAR CHECKING SOFTWARE.

The early versions of many grammar programs were primitive and not very helpful. The newer versions are much improved. Although many copy editors may not agree, this soft-

Table 31–1.   Problematic Word Pairs

while	whereas
compared to	compared with
disinterested	uninterested
since	because
that	which
complimentary	complementary
affect	effect
assure	ensure
each	every
varying	various
lay	lie

Table 31–2.   Common Problems That Copy editors Correct

Problematic Usage	*Preferred Usage*
ageing	aging
appears to be	may be
ascertained	found
assist	help
cancelled	canceled
data base	database
determine	detect, learn, find out
die from	die of
do	perform
EKG	ECG, electrocardiogram
implementing	starting
inducement	induction
Kaplan Mier method	Kaplan-Meier method
labelling	labeling
magnitude	size
many persons	many people
minimize	reduce
neurological deficit	neurologic deficit
obtundation	obtusion
of insufficient magnitude	too small
prior to	before
referred to	called
refractive	refractory
regardless of	despite
relative to	compared with
remittive	remissive
questionable utility	questionable use
the main results	the primary results
towards (British English)	toward (American English)

ware is worth using, but take the "advice" with a grain of salt. Grammatik (included as part of the Corel WordPerfect package) is excellent (see Appendix D).

PRINCIPLE 223. REWRITE SENTENCES THAT BEGIN WITH THE WORD "IT."

Compare the following sentences:

1. It was important to freeze the blood samples to ensure accurate measurements.
2. Freezing the blood samples was important to ensure accurate measurements.

Rather than starting with "it", try to guide readers through your paper by providing orientation at the beginning of sentences. For example: "In 1995, . . ." or "Among the 19 patients, ..."

Many sentences can be improved by moving the key information to the end. When possible, end sentences with a "thump" or a "bang." The last word in the sentence—and the reader's mind—receives the emphasis.

PRINCIPLE 224. USE READABLE LANGUAGE.

Buy and use a good thesaurus, such as the *Random House College Thesaurus.* Also be sure that you have an up-to-date dictionary. *Merriam-Webster's Collegiate Dictionary* is a standard used by many medical journals. The *American Heritage Dictionary of the English Language* also is helpful because it contains usage notes for problematic words (see Table 31–2).

Finally, as you edit your paper, check for phrases that could confuse readers.

As Lorraine Loviglio, who is the manager of manuscript editing at the *New England Journal of Medicine,* said: "Elegant variation has no place in medical writing. Clarity is more important." Therefore, do not alternate between "placebo group" and "control group." Use one term, and make your manuscript consistent. For example, a paper about pressure ulcers should not use the synonyms "pressure sores," "decubitus," or "bed sores."

◎ VITAL POINT

Writing does matter, and rewriting is the key. As Joseph Garland said: "There is no good medical writing—just good rewriting" (*Familiar Medical Quotations* 1968).

Now that you have finished the Editing phase, you are ready for the final phase: Revising.

P
O
W
E
R REVISING

Key Questions to Answer in the Revising Phase:

- *What needs to be improved for this paper to receive a high rating from reviewers?*

CHAPTER 32.

Revising the Final Draft

PRINCIPLE 225. PROOFREAD THE FINAL COPY OF YOUR PAPER—SEVERAL TIMES.

In the Revising phase, you should ensure that your manuscript is ready for peer review. After you finish writing and editing the final draft, read it aloud—word for word—as if someone unfamiliar with the specific subject were reading it. Be certain that your manuscript says exactly what you want it to say. For example, check that nonessential clauses, for which you lower your voice, are set off by commas. Reading your manuscript aloud helps you to evaluate the punctuation, diction, and general flow of your paper. Look for inconsistencies, such as changing from "Class" to "Stage" to "Grade." You may find it helpful to create a style sheet to record specific style points to help keep them consistent.

When you proofread your manuscript, be sure that you have not plagiarized anyone. Researchers sometimes copy sections of the Methods and Discussion sections from related reports and borrow examples from colleagues. If you use information from another source, rewrite the material in your own words or reference your sources.

PRINCIPLE 226. WATCH YOUR TENSES.

You can describe information from published work in the present tense (e.g., "X is a risk factor for Y"), the past tense (e.g., "Jones[4] demonstrated X"), or the past perfect tense (e.g., "Investigators have demonstrated X"). Describe your methods and findings in the past tense (e.g., "We found that X"), but describe your conclusions in the present tense. "We conclude that Z is a risk factor for Y, independent of X."

⊕ FOR MORE INFORMATION

For a discussion of the logic and examples of the use of tenses in medical writing, see Day (1994), or the *Publication Manual of the American Psychological Association* (APA 1994) (in Appendix D).

PRINCIPLE 227. ELIMINATE REDUNDANT SENTENCES AND NEEDLESS WORDS.

Take a red pen and see how many useless, superfluous, redundant, extra, pointless, supplementary, extraneous, additional, and excessive words you can eliminate. Also delete inappropriate or redundant sentences that were identified during your internal peer review.

For example, rather than repeating a long description of your inclusion criteria, refer to "the aforementioned criteria." Table 32–1 shows words that often can be eliminated.

In an article in the *New England Journal of Medicine,* Crichton (1975) described the most common problems with medical writing. In 1995, I surveyed experts to determine the current frequency of these problems. The results are displayed in Figures 32–1 and 32–2. As you can see, verbiage and wordiness top the list.

Table 32–1.   Unnecessary Words

Problematic Usage	Preferred Usage
an excessive number of	excessive
as the result	because
at a high risk	at high risk
at this moment in time	now
before beginning the study	before the study
data for all of the variables	data for all variables
in order to	because, to
in terms of	in, of, for
is able to	can
is know to be	is
it would appear that	apparently
Many studies have been done which support	Studies support
on the basis of	by
one of the	a
over a period of time	over time
prolonged hospital course	prolonged hospitalization
so that	so, to
that have been reported	reported
The general consensus is	The consensus is
The majority of	Most
The nutritional status	Nutritional status
small number of	few
the subsequent postoperative course	postoperative results
There are, however, no reported studies where the potential use of X has been evaluated.	We are not aware of any studies in which X has been evaluated.
this time interval	this interval
those who had given up smoking	former smokers
total number	total
was calculated by arithmetically adding	was calculated by adding
We were also able to discern a trend of higher risk of X	the risk of X was higher
which is known to be	still

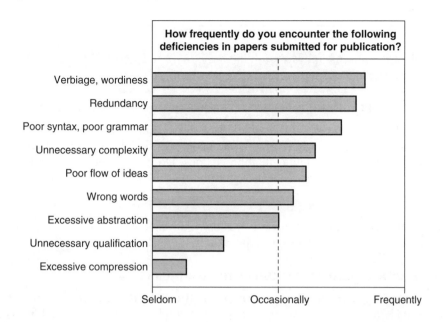

Figure 32–1. Frequency of writing problems. From question 27 of the Peer Review Questionnaire in Appendix B.

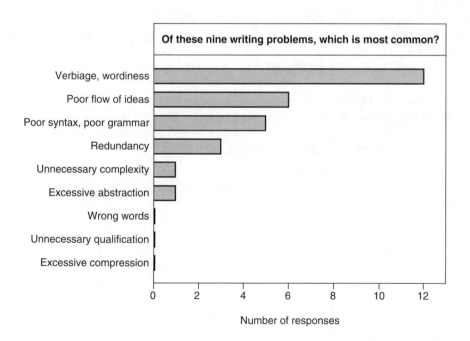

Figure 32–2. The most common writing problems. From question 28 of the Peer Review Questionnaire in Appendix B.

Pay particular attention to these problems in the Discussion to avoid the following type of comment:

> Much of the Discussion was rambling, repetitive, and somewhat conjectural.

PRINCIPLE 228. PLACE THE TABLES AND FIGURES IN THE CORRECT POSITIONS.

Place each table title at the top of the table. Place the captions for all of the figures on a single page, after the tables and before the photocopies of the glossy figures. In the captions, explain the figures and define all abbreviations. Do not put the tables and figures in the Results section; reviewers expect to find them at the end of the manuscript (see Table 12–1).

Never insert graphs in the text; reviewers consider it the sign of a dilettante. Similarly, do not use a variety of fonts (typefaces) or type sizes in the text.

PRINCIPLE 229. REMEMBER TO NUMBER THE MANUSCRIPT PAGES.

Many authors forget to number the pages of the final draft and obviously this makes a bad impression. You can print sequential numbers on pages created from different sources (e.g., a word processor and a graphics package) by following these steps:

1. Arrange the pages in the correct sequence, as described earlier, from the title page to the last figure (see Principle 44, Table 12–1).
2. On your computer, create a new file with only page numbers in the header.
3. Jump to a page number that is one higher than your manuscript's length (e.g., page 30 in a 29-page paper).
4. Type "the end" on the last page to force the computer to print the correct number of pages.
5. Load your manuscript into your printer and print the page numbers. Obviously, in the draft that you submit, do not include the page that says "the end."

PRINCIPLE 230. DOUBLE CHECK YOUR CALCULATIONS.

Use a calculator to verify that the numbers for each group total correctly. Reviewers often catch obvious mistakes this way, and if they do, they are unlikely to recommend acceptance.

CHAPTER 33.

The Cover Letter

PRINCIPLE 231. WRITE A PERSUASIVE COVER LETTER.

The cover letter is much more important than many authors realize. This letter usually is your first contact with the editor, and the editor will make some major decisions about your paper based on the contents and professionalism of your cover letter.

The purpose of the cover letter is to explain—politely—what you are submitting, and why. State the title and length of your manuscript, and indicate the number of tables and figures. Explain why you decided to submit your manuscript to that particular journal. Why would your paper be of interest to the readers of that journal? What are the strengths of your paper? Explain which section of the target journal would be most appropriate for your manuscript (e.g., Original Articles, Brief Communications, Reviews). In the salutation of the cover letter and on the envelope, make sure that you **use the current editor's name—and spell it correctly!** Avoid writing "Dear Editor."

 FOR MORE INFORMATION

Chapter 13 of *The Gregg Reference Manual* (Sabin 1993) is an excellent reference for writing a professional letter.

PRINCIPLE 232. RECOGNIZE HOW EDITORS DEFINE A GOOD ARTICLE.

Table 33–1 shows editors' definitions of a good article. If you can, include a few of these concepts in your cover letter.

PRINCIPLE 233. RECOMMEND SEVERAL REVIEWERS.

A. H. Sulzberger of the *New York Times* said: "I believe in keeping an open mind, but not so open that my brains fall out." Similarly, most reviewers try to keep an open mind. Naturally, however, some reviewers will be biased against your type of study, and getting a fair evaluation from them would be difficult.

Many journals permit—even encourage—authors to submit the names of potential reviewers, and obviously, the editor will screen out colleagues at your institution and your previous coauthors.

VITAL POINT

For some journals your paper is two to three times more likely to be accepted if it is reviewed by a recommended reviewer.

If possible, recommend a reviewer who understands your point of view, keeps an open mind, and is qualified to evaluate your paper. Remember, the first thing that some reviewers look for is whether you referenced their previous publications and whether you

Table 33–1. Editors' Definitions of a Good Article*

Good Study Design

- Clean methodology
- One that develops a creative or original problem derived from a strong theoretical base; clear hypotheses, adequate sample size, with conclusions drawn specifically from the findings
- Well designed
- Good statistics (fitted to problem type and size)
- Strict adherence to scientific and statistical methodology
- Adequate data sets with clinical correlation
- One that reports clearly and in sufficient detail on a well-designed and well-conducted research experiment or an important question

Original and Important Results

- New information
- Clinically useful
- Broad clinical application
- Well designed, addressing a new idea, not too long, incisive and informative Discussion
- Exciting, new, well-supported data
- Original study, with well-defined aims; well conceived, executed, and presented
- Newness, trueness, and timeliness

Strong Presentation of the Data

- Clearly presented
- Targets readership
- Organized, logical, clearly written, with good Methods
- Well referenced
- One that conforms to the journal's information for authors and contains new, important, well set out information that is likely to really interest readers; refers to up-to-date, relevant references in the world literature

Conclusions Supported by Data

- Results not overinterpreted
- Appropriate interpretation of results

Well-written and Concise

- Short, concise, clean methodology

(continued)

Table 33–1. Editors' Definitions of a Good Article* (*continued*)
• A concise, well-written report of a well-designed study • Good writing • One that has content that meets the journal's purpose and is well written (readable) • Good flow of ideas; easy to follow • Useful information that is well written
* From question 30 of the Peer Review Questionnaire in Appendix B.

commented favorably on their findings. You can avoid insulting the recommended reviewers by including their relevant publications in your references, but be careful to stay within ethical boundaries.

Further, let the editor know whether there is anyone you do not want to review your paper. Editors usually honor these requests. You also can ask to have reviewers "blinded" to the authors' identities.

PRINCIPLE 234. BE CANDID ABOUT WHAT INFORMATION IN YOUR PAPER HAS BEEN PUBLISHED OR PRESENTED BEFORE.

Reassure the editor that the information in your paper has not been published before. Also state that you will not submit the manuscript to another journal until the review process is complete.

Be sure to describe and submit a copy of any part of the research that has been published (e.g., the abstract). Also tell the editor about any closely related papers, but then explain what NEW information this paper provides.

PRINCIPLE 235. PROVIDE A CONTACT PERSON.

On the title page and in the cover letter, identify the author who is responsible for manuscript negotiations. Provide the corresponding author's full name and full mailing address, all pertinent telephone numbers, a fax number, and if applicable, an E-mail address. Make sure that the address is clear and complete, especially if it is outside the United States. You also may want to ask the editor to return the glossy prints of the figures to the contact person if the manuscript is not accepted.

PRINCIPLE 236. INTRODUCE YOURSELF AND YOUR COAUTHORS TO THE EDITOR—POLITELY.

Although few authors do this, you should be aware that providing information about yourself and your coauthors can be helpful at some journals; at others, it makes no difference. In your cover letter, you can briefly provide information, such as your credentials and the experience that makes you uniquely qualified to write this paper. Although you may have explained in the Methods section where the study was conducted, in the cover letter, you can explain the advantages of conducting a study there.

Explain that each coauthor has seen and approved the final draft of the manuscript. See the section "Requirements for the Submission of Manuscripts" in Appendix A.

Although a well-written cover letter is helpful, a more important concern, as one expert said, is "to have the correct format, proper number of copies, correct ordering of contents of the manuscript, and enclosed copies of glossy prints of pictures. Photocopies, rather than glossy prints, of certain figures are often difficult for reviewers to interpret and can lead to the rejection of that manuscript."

Finally, never staple the pages of the cover letter or manuscript. Use a paper clip.

CHAPTER 34.

Responding to Peer Reviewers' Comments

PRINCIPLE 237. RECOGNIZE HOW THE JOURNAL REVIEW AND DECISION-MAKING PROCESS WORKS.

Peer reviewers often spend considerable time and effort evaluating manuscripts. Ordinarily, they are not compensated for this work. Most reviewers give extensive thought to improving the papers that are submitted for publication, so be diplomatic and demonstrate your knowledge of how the system operates.

If your manuscript is returned with comments from reviewers, make those changes that will improve the paper. However, it is essential to address all the comments in your revised manuscript.

 VITAL POINT

If the reviewers recommend some changes that you disagree with, explain your reasons for disagreement in the cover letter. Do not simply say: "I disagree."

Good reasons for not making recommended changes include invalid criticisms and unavailable data. If you strongly disagree with a reviewer's point, do not make the change, but consider adding an explanation or clarification in your paper for the many readers who will ask the same question.

Return a photocopy of the reviewers' comments, with each point addressed. Detail the changes that you made (e.g., "Reviewer 1, page 6, line 17—NS was changed to '$P = 0.06$.'").

An invitation to resubmit your paper does not guarantee that it will be accepted. You must address the concerns of the reviewers to their satisfaction. Do not cavalierly ignore their suggestions and imply that they are beneath you.

Some reviewers may ask you to obtain more information or perform more detailed analysis. Sometimes this situation occurs when a reviewer merely is abusing his power, rather than demonstrating his expertise. Carefully consider all of the reviewers' comments, and as long as the recommended changes do not detract from your paper, follow their suggestions.

Editors understand that reviewers may be biased and that authors may be unresponsive to their comments. Sometimes you can ease the situation simply by talking on the telephone with the editor. Most editors are reasonable people with whom you can discuss your concerns. Remember, editors want to help you publish a clear, concise, and accurate paper.

PRINCIPLE 238. FOLLOW THE SUGGESTIONS FOR RESUBMITTING
YOUR PAPER.

Table 34–1 shows suggestions for resubmitting a paper.

PRINCIPLE 239. DO NOT BE DISCOURAGED BY CRITICISM.

Nearly every published manuscript has been revised based on peer reviewers' comments. Of course, articles invited by the editor have a high probability of publication, but unsolicited manuscripts rarely are accepted outright by three reviewers and an editor.

PRINCIPLE 240. REVISE YOUR MANUSCRIPT BEFORE YOU SUBMIT IT TO
ANOTHER JOURNAL.

If your manuscript is rejected, revise it promptly and submit it to another journal—before you lose your momentum and your research team. Although many prestigious medical journals reject more than 90% of submitted manuscripts, 80% of the rejected manuscripts are published elsewhere. Of the papers that are published elsewhere, 20% of authors make the mistake of never changing the flaws that were pointed out by the first journal's reviewers. Find the energy to avoid being among this 20% of authors.

Remember that you are responsible for finding and correcting the flaws in your paper. Your paper may contain some information that led reviewers to misunderstand your study and criticize it unfairly. However, the next journal that you submit your paper to may send your paper to the same reviewer as the first journal. If you do not make any of the recommended changes, you may receive the same critique and rejection.

Table 34–1.   Suggestions for Resubmitting Your Revised Manuscript

1. Follow the suggestions of the reviewers and editors, and make all (or most) of the suggested changes.
2. Do not make changes that are simply cosmetic.
3. Obtain approval from each coauthor for all changes.
4. Explain in detail what you have done. Answer each point of the critique and include the page, paragraph, and sentence number for the original and revised manuscripts in the answer.
5. Label, date, and return both the original and the revised manuscripts.
6. Include the manuscript number in your letter and on the revised version.
7. Respond promptly.

If your manuscript was rejected, remember that unless the editor has given you some real encouragement, in most cases, you are wasting your time by sending your manuscript back to the editor for reconsideration. Even if you make all of the changes suggested by the reviewers, they are unlikely to change their minds, and your project may be delayed for months.

PRINCIPLE 241. UNDERSTAND HOW PUBLISHING DECISIONS ARE REACHED.

Many inexperienced medical researchers mistakenly believe that peer reviewers decide whether to accept or reject a manuscript. Many reviewers also believe that they have this authority. For most journals, however, the editor-in-chief makes the final decision. This distinction is important because reviewers and editors often give numerical scores to different features of a paper (see Figure 28–1). These scores are weighted and summed, to rank potential manuscripts. Papers with the highest scores are considered for publication. The rating system often includes categories such as those shown in Table 34–2. Some journal editors ask reviewers to complete a simple evaluation form, such as that shown in Figure 34–1. Whichever system is used, your chances of acceptance increase if you consider the perspective of reviewers and editors.

Most journals receive more than four times as many papers as they can publish. Although many papers represent sound work, they are rejected because they do not receive a high enough ranking. Because reviewers typically give papers numerical scores and not simply a pass or fail grade, many trivial errors can lower a paper's score to below the threshold for acceptance. Many researchers believe that their paper will not be rejected because of minor imperfections. This is simply not true.

PRINCIPLE 242. RECOGNIZE PROBLEMS INHERENT IN THE PEER REVIEW PROCESS.

As one reviewer observed:

> The peer review process is imperfect and only works because nobody has a better way. I've had some incredibly stupid reviews indicating the reviewer hadn't read or hadn't understood the thrust of the paper. Another frequent problem is when reviewers ask for conflicting changes. What can you do about that? The whole process is rather complicated, often leading to unwarranted rejection of important, but negative, results and innovative, but unorthodox, reports.

Table 34–2.   Typical Elements in a Priority Rating System
Clinical and scientific quality
Timeliness of the subject matter
Perceived reader needs
Peer reviewer comments
General editorial requirements

1. Quality

    ☐ Superior

    ☐ Good

    ☐ Fair

    ☐ Poor

2. Recommendation for publication

    ☐ Accept

    ☐ Accept with minor revision

    ☐ Major revision; reconsider

    ☐ Reject because of:

        ☐ Unimportant topic

        ☐ Unwarranted conclusions

        ☐ Adequate coverage of subject in the literature already

        ☐ Poor organization

3. Recommended priority for publication if major criticisms are satisfied

    ☐ Highest priority

    ☐ Intermediate priority

    ☐ Lowest priority

    ☐ Criticisms probably cannot be satisfied.

Figure 34–1. Typical reviewer's evaluation form.

Proofreaders' Marks

Instruction	Mark in margin	Mark on proof	Corrected type
General			
Delete	ℰ	the ~~good~~ word	the word
Delete and close up space	ℰ̣	the wo**o**rd	the word
Insert indicated material	*good*	the⌃word	the good word
Let it stand	(stet)	the ~~good~~ word	the good word
Spell out	(sp)	②words	two words
Paragraphing			
New paragraph	¶	"Where is it?"⌐ "It's on the shelf." ⌃	"Where is it?" "It's on the shelf."
Flush paragraph	▯¶	"Where is it?"⌐ "It's on the shelf." ⌃	"Where is it?" "It's on the shelf."
Position and spacing			
Transpose	(tr)	the⟮word⟯good	the good word:
Move left	⊏	⊏ the word	the word
Move right	⊐	⊐the word	the word
Move down	⊔	⊔the⟍word	the word
Move up	⊓	⌐the⟍word	the word
Align	‖	‖ the word the word	the word the word
Straighten line	＝	‾the word	the word
Insert space	#	the⟍word	the word
Equalize space	(eq #)	the⌃good⌃word	the good word
Close up	⌒	the wo⌒rd	the word
en space	⎅/N	⌃the word	the word
em space	⎅/M	⌃the word	the word
Punctuation			
period	⊙	This is the word⌃	This is the word
comma	⋀	words⌃words, words	words, words, words
hyphen	＝⌃	word⌃for⌃word test	word-for-word test
colon	(:)	The following words⌃	The following words:
semicolon	⋀>	Scan the words/skim the words. ⌃	Scan the words; skim the words.
apostrophe	⌄∨	John⌄s words	John's words
double quotation marks	∨/∨	the word⌃word∨	the word "word"
single quotation marks	∨/∨	the "good⌃word⌃"	the "good 'word'"
brackets	E / ∃	He read from the Word ⌃in the Bible⌃	He read from the Word [in the Bible].
en dash	⤶N	1964⌃1972	1964–1972
em dash	⤶M	The dictionary⌃how often it is needed⌃ belongs in every home	The dictionary—how often it is needed— belongs in every home
asterisk	∨*	word∨	word*
dagger	∨†	a word⌃	a word†
double dagger	∨‡	words and words⌃	words and words‡
section symbol	§	⌃Book Reviews	§Book Reviews
virgule (slash)	/	either/or	either/or
three ellipses	⎮O⎮O⎮O⎮	the⌃word	the...word
four ellipses	⌒O⎮O⎮O⎮O⎮	the word⌃	the word....
Style of type			
uppercase	(uc)	the word	The Word
lowercase	(lc)	The Word	the word
small capitals	(sc)	the word	THE WORD
italic	(ital)	the entry word	the entry *word*
roman	(rom)	the entry (word)	the entry word
boldface	(bf)	the entry word	the entry **word**
lightface	(lf)	(the entry word)	the entry word
superior	∨2	2∨=4	2²=4
inferior	⋀2	H₂0	H₂O

Figure 34–2. Standard proofreaders' marks. Copyright © 1993 by Houghton Mifflin Company. Reproduced by permission from *The American Heritage Dictionary of the English Language, Third Edition.*

Table 34–3.   Examples of Ideal Papers

- Most articles by Leonard Seeff (e.g., Seeff et al. 1992)
- Some of the work by Haynes and Sackett (e.g., Sackett et al. 1991; Sackett 1979)
- "Strategies for the Analysis of Oncogene Overexpression": Studies of the *neu* Oncogene in Breast Carcinoma" (Naber et al. 1990)
- "A Controlled Trial of Antepartum Glucocorticoid Treatment for Prevention of the Respiratory Distress Syndrome in Premature Infants" (Liggins and Howie 1972)
- "The Effect of Vitamin E and Beta Carotene on the Incidence of Lung Cancer and Other Cancers in Male Smokers" (Alpha-Tocopherol, Beta Carotene Cancer Prevention Study Group 1994; Marantz 1994)
- "Standardized Nerve Conduction Studies in the Lower Limb of the Healthy Elderly" (Falco et al. 1994)
- "Hemodynamic Changes in the Early Postburn Patient: The Influence of Fluid Administration and of a Vasodilator (Hydralazine)" (Pruitt, Mason, and Moncrief 1971)
- We are still searching for the "ideal" paper!

THE FINAL STEPS

PRINCIPLE 243. CHECK THE GALLEY PROOFS OR PAGE PROOFS CAREFULLY.

If your paper is accepted, carefully proofread the version that the publisher sends to you. **Also insist that each coauthor check the proof carefully.** Depending on your institution, you also may want to show a copy to the public relations department.

Never make major changes at this point.

Send your changes to the editor promptly. Editors often ask authors to return proofs within 48 hours. Despite the time limitations, devoting enough time to check for typographical errors, incorrect P values, and spelling and grammatical errors is a crucial part of producing a quality paper. Because tables often require substantial reformatting, check the tables in the proofs against your originals. If you used any "in press" papers as references, update them by providing the volume, year, and page numbers. If you used any abstracts as references, determine whether they have been published as full papers, and if so, update your citations.

Communicating with the copy editor is essential at this point. Always return the proofs, even if you do not wish to make any changes. If you do not understand any marks or queries, see Figure 34–2 or call the copy editor to resolve the problem.

PRINCIPLE 244. STUDY "IDEAL" PAPERS.

Because the focus of this book is avoiding problems, I want to end with some positive models. Editors and reviewers provided the responses and examples of "ideal" papers shown in Table 34–3. Another source of positive models is the book "One Hundred Years of JAMA Landmark Articles," available from the AMA.

PRINCIPLE 245. KNOW WHEN TO STOP.

Finally, remember that a good paper "has a definite structure, makes its point and then shuts up" (Lock 1991).

1. Uniform Requirements for Manuscripts Submitted to Biomedical Journals

*International Committee of Medical Journal Editors**

A small group of editors of general medical journals met informally in Vancouver, British Columbia, in 1978 to establish guidelines for the format of manuscripts submitted to their journals. The group became known as the Vancouver Group. Its requirements for manuscripts, including formats for bibliographic references developed by the National Library of Medicine, were first published in 1979. The Vancouver Group expanded and evolved into the International Committee of Medical Journal Editors (ICMJE), which meets annually; gradually it has broadened its concerns.

The committee has produced five editions of the "Uniform Requirements for Manuscripts Submitted to Biomedical Journals." Over the years, issues have arisen that go beyond manuscript preparation. Some of these issues are now covered in the "Uniform Requirements"; others are addressed in separate statements. Each statement has been published in a scientific journal.

The fifth edition (1997) is an effort to reorganize and reword the fourth edition to increase clarity and address concerns about rights, privacy, descriptions of methods, and other matters. The total content of "Uniform Requirements for Manuscripts Submitted to Biomedical Journals" may be reproduced for educational, not-for-profit purposes without regard for copyright; the committee encourages distribution of the material.

Journals that agree to use the "Uniform Requirements" (over 500 do so) are asked to cite the 1997 document in their instructions to authors. Inquiries and comments should be sent to Kathleen Case at the ICMJE secretariat office, *Annals of Internal Medicine,* American College of Physicians, Independence Mall W., Sixth St. at Race, Philadelphia, PA 19106–1572, United States (Phone: 215–351–2661; Fax: 215–351–2644; e-mail: kathyc@acp.mhs.compuserve.com).

Publications represented on the ICMJE in 1996 were: the *Annuals of Internal Medicine,* the *British Medical Journal,* the *Canadian Medical Association Journal,* the *Journal of the American Medical Association,* the *Lancet,* the *Medical Journal of Australia,* the *New England Journal of Medicine,* the *New Zealand Medical Journal,* the *Tidsskrift for den Norske Laegeforening,* the *Western Journal of Medicine,* and the *Index Medicus.*

It is important to emphasize what these requirements do and do not imply.

First, the "Uniform Requirements" are instructions to authors on how to prepare manuscripts, not to editors on publication style. (But many journals have drawn on them for elements of their publication styles.)

Second, if authors prepare their manuscripts in the style specified in these requirements, editors of the participating journals will not return the manuscripts for changes in

---

*Members of the Committee are Linda Hawes Clever, *Western Journal of Medicine;* Lois Ann Colaianni, *Index Medicus;* Frank Davidoff, *Annals of Internal Medicine;* Richard Glass, *JAMA;* Richard Horton, *Lancet;* Jerome P. Kassier and Marcia Angell, *New England Journal of Medicine;* George Lundberg and Richard Glass, *JAMA;* Magne Nylenna, *Tidsskrift for Den Norske Legeforening;* Richard G. Robinson, *New Zealand Medical Journal;* Richard Smith, *BMJ;* Bruce P. Squires, *Canadian Medical Association Journal;* Robert Utiger, *The New England Journal of Medicine;* Martin Van-Der Weyden, *The Medical Journal of Australia;* and Patricia Woolf, *Princeton University.*

Reprinted with permission from the International Committee of Medical Journal Editors.

style before considering them for publication. In the publishing process, however, the journals may alter accepted manuscripts to conform with details of their publication styles.

Third, authors sending manuscripts to a participating journal should not try to prepare them in accordance with the publication style of that journal but should follow the "Uniform Requirements."

Authors must also follow the instructions to authors in the journal as to what topics are suitable for that journal and the types of papers that may be submitted—for example, original articles, reviews, or case reports. In addition, the journal's instructions are likely to contain other requirements unique to that journal, such as the number of copies of a manuscript that are required, acceptable languages, length of articles, and approved abbreviations.

Participating journals are expected to state in their instructions to authors that their requirements are in accordance with the "Uniform Requirements for Manuscripts Submitted to Biomedical Journals" and to cite a published version.

ISSUES TO CONSIDER BEFORE SUBMITTING A MANUSCRIPT

Redundant or Duplicate Publication

Redundant or duplicate publication is publication of a paper that overlaps substantially with one already published.

Readers of primary source periodicals deserve to be able to trust that what they are reading is original unless there is a clear statement that the article is being republished by the choice of the author and editor. The bases of this position are international copyright laws, ethical conduct, and cost-effective use of resources.

Most journals do not wish to receive papers on work that has already been reported in large part in a published article or is contained in another paper that has been submitted or accepted for publication elsewhere, in print or in electronic media. This policy does not preclude the journal considering a paper that has been rejected by another journal, or a complete report that follows publication of a preliminary report, such as an abstract or poster displayed for colleagues at a professional meeting. Nor does it prevent journals considering a paper that has been presented at a scientific meeting but not published in full or that is being considered for publication in a proceedings or similar format. Press reports of scheduled meetings will not usually be regarded as breaches of this rule, but such reports should not be amplified by additional data or copies of tables and illustrations.

When submitting a paper, the author should always make a full statement to the editor about all submissions and previous reports that might be regarded as redundant or duplicate publication of the same or very similar work. The author should alert the editor if the work includes subjects about which a previous report has been published. Any such work should be referred to and referenced in the new paper. Copies of such material should be included with the submitted paper to help the editor decide how to handle the matter.

If redundant or duplicate publication is attempted or occurs without such notification, authors should expect editorial action to be taken. At the least, prompt rejection of the submitted manuscript should be expected. If the editor was not aware of the violations and the article has already been published, then a notice of redundant or duplicate publication will probably be published with or without the author's explanation or approval.

Preliminary release, usually to public media, of scientific information described in a paper that has been accepted but not yet published violates the policies of many journals. In a few cases, and only by arrangement with the editor, preliminary release of data may be acceptable—for example, if there is a public health emergency.

Acceptable Secondary Publication

Secondary publication in the same or another language, especially in other countries, is justifiable, and can be beneficial, provided all of the following conditions are met:

- The authors have received approval from the editors of both journals; the editor concerned with secondary publication must have a photocopy, reprint, or manuscript of the primary version.
- The priority of the primary publication is respected by a publication interval of at least one week (unless specifically negotiated otherwise by both editors).
- The paper for secondary publication is intended for a different group of readers; an abbreviated version could be sufficient.
- The secondary version faithfully reflects the data and interpretations of the primary version.
- The footnote on the title page of the secondary version informs readers, peers, and documenting agencies that the paper has been published in whole or in part and states the primary reference. A suitable footnote might read: "This article is based on a study first reported in the [title of journal, with full reference]."

  Permission for such secondary publication should be free of charge.

Protection of Patients' Rights to Privacy

Patients have a right to privacy that should not be infringed without informed consent. Identifying information should not be published in written descriptions, photographs, and pedigrees unless the information is essential for scientific purposes and the patient (or parent or guardian) gives written informed consent for publication. Informed consent for this purpose requires that the patient be shown the manuscript to be published.

Identifying details should be omitted if they are not essential, but patient data should never be altered or falsified in an attempt to attain anonymity. Complete anonymity is difficult to achieve, and informed consent should be obtained if there is any doubt. For example, masking the eye region in photographs of patients is inadequate protection of anonymity.

The requirement for informed consent should be included in the journal's instructions for authors. When informed consent has been obtained it should be indicated in the published article.

REQUIREMENTS FOR THE SUBMISSION OF MANUSCRIPTS

Summary of Technical Requirements

- Double space all parts of manuscripts.
- Begin each section or component on a new page.
- Review the sequence: title page, abstract and key words, text, acknowledgments, references, tables (each on separate page), legends.
- Illustrations, unmounted prints, should be no larger than 203×254 mm (8×10 inches).
- Include permission to reproduce previously published material or to use illustrations that may identify human subjects.
- Enclose transfer of copyright and other forms.
- Submit required number of paper copies.
- Keep copies of everything submitted.

Preparation of Manuscript

The text of observational and experimental articles is usually (but not necessarily) divided into sections with the headings Introduction, Methods, Results, and Discussion. Long articles may need subheadings within some sections (especially the Results and Discussion sections) to clarify their content. Other types of articles, such as case reports, reviews, and editorials, are likely to need other formats. Authors should consult individual journals for further guidance.

Type or print out the manuscript on white bond paper, 216×279 mm (8.5×11 inches), or ISO A4 (212×297 mm), with margins of at least 25 mm (1 inch). Type or print on only one side of the paper. Use double-spacing throughout, including for the title page, abstract, text, acknowledgments, references, individual tables, and legends. Number pages consecutively, beginning with the title page. Put the page number in the upper or lower right-hand corner of each page.

Manuscripts on Disks

For papers that are close to final acceptance, some journals require authors to provide a copy in electronic form (on a disk); they may accept a variety of word-processing formats or text (ASCII) files.

When submitting disks, authors should:

- Be certain to include a printout of the version of the article that is on the disk;
- Put only the latest version of the manuscript on the disk
- Name the file clearly;
- Label the disk with the format of the file and the file name;
- Provide information on the hardware and software used.

Authors should consult the journal's instructions to authors for acceptable formats, conventions for naming files, number of copies to be submitted, and other details.

Title Page

The title page should carry 1) the title of the article, which should be concise but informative; 2) the name by which each author is known, with his or her highest academic degree(s) and institutional affiliation; 3) the name of the department(s) and institution(s) to which the work should be attributed; 4) disclaimers, if any; 5) the name and address of the author responsible for correspondence about the manuscript; 6) the name and address of the author to whom requests for reprints should be addressed or a statement that reprints will not be available from the authors; 7) source(s) of support in the form of grants, equipment, drugs, or all of these; and 8) a short running head or footline of no more than 40 characters (count letters and spaces) at the foot of the title page.

Authorship

All persons designated as authors should qualify for authorship. Each author should have participated sufficiently in the work to take public responsibility for the content.

Authorship credit should be based only on substantial contributions to 1) conception and design, or analysis and interpretation of data; and to 2) drafting the article or revising it critically for important intellectual content; and on 3) final approval of the version to be published. Conditions 1, 2, and 3 must all be met. Participation solely in the acquisition of funding or the collection of data does not justify authorship. General supervision of the research group is not sufficient for authorship. Any part of an article critical to its main conclusions must be the responsibility of at least one author.

Editors may ask authors to describe what each contributed; this information may be published.

Increasingly, multicenter trials are attributed to a corporate author. All members of the group who are named as authors, either in the authorship position below the title or in a footnote, should fully meet the above criteria for authorship. Group members who do not meet these criteria should be listed, with their permission, in the Acknowledgments or in an appendix (see Acknowledgments).

The order of authorship should be a joint decision of the coauthors. Because the order is assigned in different ways, its meaning cannot be inferred accurately unless it is stated by the authors. Authors may wish to explain the order of authorship in a footnote. In deciding on the order, authors should be aware that many journals limit the number of authors listed in the table of contents and that the U.S. National Library of Medicine (NLM) lists in MEDLINE only the first 24 plus the last author when there are more than 25 authors.

Abstract and Key Words

The second page should carry an abstract (of no more than 150 words for unstructured abstracts or 250 words for structured abstracts). The abstract should state the purposes of the study or investigation, basic procedures (selection of study subjects or laboratory animals; observational and analytical methods), main findings (giving specific data and their statistical significance, if possible), and the principal conclusions. It should emphasize new and important aspects of the study or observations.

Below the abstract authors should provide, and identify as such, 3 to 10 key words or short phrases that will assist indexers in cross-indexing the article and may be published with the abstract. Terms from the Medical Subject Headings (MeSH) list of *Index Medicus* should be used; if suitable MeSH terms not yet available for recently introduced terms, present terms may be used.

Introduction

State the purpose of the article and summarize the rationale for the study or observation. Give only strictly pertinent references and do not include data or conclusions from the work being reported.

Methods

Describe your selection of the observational or experimental subjects (patients or laboratory animals, including controls) clearly. Identify the age, sex, and other important characteristics of the subjects. The definition and relevance of race and ethnicity are ambiguous. Authors should be particularly careful about using these categories.

Identify the methods, apparatus (give the manufacturer's name and address in parentheses), and procedures in sufficient detail to allow other workers to reproduce the results. Give references to established methods, including statistical methods (see below); provide references and brief descriptions for methods that have been published but are not well known; describe new or substantially modified methods, give reasons for using them, and evaluate their limitations. Identify precisely all drugs and chemicals used, including generic name(s), dose(s), and route(s) of administration.

Reports of randomized clinical trials should present information on all major study elements, including the protocol (study population, interventions or exposures, out-comes, and the rationale for statistical analysis), assignment of interventions (methods of randomization, concealment of allocation to treatment groups), and the method of mask-ing (blinding).

Authors submitting review manuscripts should include a section describing the methods used for locating, selecting, extracting, and synthesizing data. These methods should also be summarized in the abstract.

Ethics

When reporting experiments on human subjects, indicate whether the procedures fol-lowed were in accordance with the ethical standards of the responsible committee on hu-man experimentation (institutional or regional) and with the Helsinki Declaration of 1975, as revised in 1983. Do not use patients' names, initials, or hospital numbers, espe-cially in illustrative material. When reporting experiments on animals, indicate whether the institution's or a national research council's guide for, or any national law on, the care and use of laboratory animals was followed.

Statistics

Describe statistical methods with enough detail to enable a knowledgeable reader with access to the original data to verify the reported results. When possible, quantify find-ings and present them with appropriate indicators of measurement error or uncertainty (such as confidence intervals). Avoid relying solely on statistical hypothesis testing, such as the use of P values, which fails to convey important quantitative information. Discuss the eligibility of experimental subjects. Give details about randomization. Describe the methods for and success of any blinding of observations. Report complications of treat-ment. Give numbers of observations. Report losses to observation (such as dropouts from a clinical trial). References for the design of the study and statistical methods should be to standard works when possible (with pages stated) rather than to papers in which the designs or methods were originally reported. Specify any general-use com-puter programs used.

Put a general description of methods in the Methods section. When data are sum-marized in the Results section, specify the statistical methods used to analyze them. Re-strict tables and figures to those needed to explain the argument of the paper and to as-sess its support. Use graphs as an alternative to tables with many entries; do not duplicate data in graphs and tables. Avoid nontechnical uses of technical terms in statistics, such as "random" (which implies a randomizing device), "normal," "significant," "correlations," and "sample." Define statistical terms, abbreviations, and most symbols.

Results

Present your results in logical sequence in the text, tables, and illustrations. Do not re-peat in the text all the data in the tables or illustrations; emphasize or summarize only im-portant observations.

Discussion

Emphasize the new and important aspects of the study and the conclusions that follow from them. Do not repeat in detail data or other material given in the Introduction or the Results section. Include in the Discussion section the implications of the findings and their limitations, including implications for future research. Relate the observations to other relevant studies.

Link the conclusions with the goals of the study but avoid unqualified statements and conclusions not completely supported by the data. In particular, authors should avoid making statements on economic benefits and costs unless their manuscript includes economic data and analysis. Avoid claiming priority and alluding to work that has not been completed. State new hypotheses when warranted, but clearly label them as such. Recommendations, when appropriate, may be included.

Acknowledgments

At an appropriate place in the article (the title-page footnote or an appendix to the text; see the journal's requirements), one or more statements should specify 1) contributions that need acknowledging but do not justify authorship, such as general support by a departmental chair; 2) acknowledgments of technical help; 3) acknowledgments of financial and material support, which should specify the nature of the support; and 4) relationships that may pose a conflict of interest.

Persons who have contributed intellectually to the paper but whose contributions do not justify authorship may be named and their function or contribution described—for example, "scientific adviser," "critical review of study proposal," "data collection," or "participation in clinical trial." Such persons must have given their permission to be named. Authors are responsible for obtaining written permission from persons acknowledged by name, because readers may infer their endorsement of the data and conclusions.

Technical help should be acknowledged in a paragraph separate from that acknowledging other contributions.

References

References should be numbered consecutively in the order in which they are first mentioned in the text. Identify references in text, tables, and legends by Arabic numerals in parentheses. References cited only in tables or figure legends should be numbered in accordance with the sequence established by the first identification in the text of the particular table or figure.

Use the style of the examples below, which are based on the formats used by the NLM in *Index Medicus*. The titles of journals should be abbreviated according to the style used in *Index Medicus*. Consult the List of Journals Indexed in *Index Medicus*, published annually as a separate publication by the library and as a list in the January issue of *Index Medicus*. The list can also be obtained through the library's web site (http://www.nlm.nih.gov).

Avoid using abstracts as references. References to papers accepted but not yet published should be designated as "in press" or "forthcoming"; authors should obtain written permission to cite such papers as well as verification that they have been accepted for publication. Information from manuscripts submitted but not accepted should be cited in the text as "unpublished observations" with written permission from the source.

Avoid citing a "personal communication" unless it provides essential information not available from a public source, in which case the name of the person and date of communication should be cited in parentheses in the text. For scientific articles, authors should obtain written permission and confirmation of accuracy from the source of a personal communication.

The references must be verified by the author(s) against the original documents.

The Uniform Requirements style (the Vancouver style) is based largely on an ANSI standard style adapted by the NLM for its databases. Notes have been added where Vancouver style differs from the style now used by NLM.

Articles in Journals

1. *Standard journal article*
   List the first six authors followed by et al. (Note: NLM now lists up to 25 authors; if there are more than 25 authors, NLM lists the first 24, then the last author, then et al.)

   > Vega KJ, Pina I, Krevsky B. Heart transplantation is associated with an increased risk for pancreatobiliary disease. Ann Intern Med 1996 Jun 1;124 (11):980–3.

   As an option, if a journal carries continuous pagination throughout a volume (as many medical journals do), the month and issue number may be omitted. (Note: For consistency, the option is used throughout the examples in "Uniform Requirements". NLM does not use the option.)

   > Vega KJ, Pina I, Krevsky B. Heart transplantation is associated with an increased risk for pancreatobiliary disease. Ann Intern Med 1996;124:980–3.

   More than six authors:

   > Parkin DM, Clayton D, Black RJ, Masuyer E, Friedl HP, Ivanov E, et al. Childhood leukaemia in Europe after Chernobyl: 5 year follow-up. Br J Cancer 1996;73:1006–12.

2. *Organization as author*

   > The Cardiac Society of Australia and New Zealand. Clinical exercise stress testing. Safety and performance guidelines. Med J Aust 1996; 164: 282–4.

3. *No author given*

   > Cancer in South Africa [editorial]. S Afr Med J 1994;84:15.

4. *Article not in English*
   (Note: NLM translates the title to English, encloses the translation in square brackets, and adds an abbreviated language designator.)

   > Ryder TE, Haukeland EA, Solhaug JH. Bilateral infrapatellar seneruptur hostidligere frisk kvinne. Tidsskr Nor Laegeforen 1996;116:41–2.

5. *Volume with supplement*

   > Shen HM, Zhang QF. Risk assessment of nickel carcinogenicity and occupational lung cancer. Environ Health Perspect 1994;102 Suppl 1:275–82.

6. *Issue with supplement*

   > Payne DK, Sullivan MD, Massie MJ. Women's psychological reactions to breast cancer. Semin Oncol 1996;23(1 Suppl 2):89–97.

7. *Volume with part*

   > Ozben T, Nacitarhan S, Tuncer N. Plasma and urine sialic acid in non-insulin dependent diabetes mellitus. Ann Clin Biochem 1995;32(Pt 3):303–6.

8. *Issue with part*

   > Poole GH, Mills SM. One hundred consecutive cases of flap lacerations of the leg in ageing patients. N Z Med J 1994;107(986 Pt 1):377–8.

9. *Issue with no volume*

Turan I, Wredmark T, Fellander-Tsai L. Arthroscopic ankle arthrodesis in rheumatoid arthritis. Clin Orthop 1995;(320):110–4.

10. *No issue or volume*

Browell DA, Lennard TW. Immunologic status of the cancer patient and the effects of blood transfusion on antitumor responses. Curr Opin Gen Surg 1993:325–33.

11. *Pagination in Roman numerals*

Fisher GA, Sikic BI. Drug resistance in clinical oncology and hematology. Introduction. Hematol Oncol Clin North Am 1995 Apr; 9(2):xi–xii.

12. *Type of article indicated as needed*

Enzensberger W, Fischer PA. Metronome in Parkinson's disease [letter]. Lancet 1996;347:1337. Clement J, De Bock R. Hematological complications of hantavirus nephropathy (HVN) [abstract]. Kidney Int 1992;42:1285.

13. *Article containing retraction*

Garey CE, Schwarzman AL, Rise ML, Seyfried TN. Ceruloplasmin gene defect associated with epilepsy in EL mice [retraction of Garey CE, Schwarzman AL, Rise ML, Seyfried TN. In: Nat Genet 1994;6:426–31]. Nat Genet 1995;11:104.

14. *Article retracted*

Liou GI, Wang M, Matragoon S. Precocious IRBP gene expression during mouse development [retracted in Invest Ophthalmol Vis Sci 1994;35:3127]. Invest Ophthalmol Vis Sci 1994;35:1083–8.

15. *Article with published erratum*

Hamlin JA, Kahn AM. Herniography in symptomatic patients following inguinal hernia repair [published erratum appears in West J Med 1995;162:278]. West J Med 1995;162:28–31.

Books and Other Monographs

(Note: Previous Vancouver style incorrectly had a comma rather than a semicolon between the publisher and the date.)

16. *Personal author(s)*

Ringsven MK, Bond D. Gerontology and leadership skills for nurses. 2nd ed. Albany (NY): Delmar Publishers; 1996.

17. *Editor(s), compiler(s) as author*

Norman IJ, Redfern SJ, editors. Mental health care for elderly people. New York: Churchill Livingstone; 1996.

18. *Organization as author and publisher*

Institute of Medicine (US). Looking at the future of the Medicaid program. Washington: The Institute; 1992.

19. *Chapter in a book*

(Note: Previous Vancouver style had a colon rather than a p before pagination.)

Phillips SJ, Whisnant JP. Hypertension and stroke. In: Laragh JH, Brenner BM, editors. Hypertension: pathophysiology, diagnosis, and management. 2nd ed. New York: Raven Press; 1995. p. 465–78.

20. *Conference proceedings*

   Kimura J, Shibasaki H, editors. Recent advances in clinical neurophysiology. Proceedings of the 10th International Congress of EMG and Clinical Neurophysiology; 1995 Oct 15–19; Kyoto, Japan. Amsterdam: Elsevier; 1996.

21. *Conference paper*

   Bengtsson S, Solheim BG. Enforcement of data protection, privacy and security in medical informatics. In: Lun KC, Degoulet P, Piemme TE, Rienhoff O, editors. MEDINFO 92. Proceedings of the 7th World Congress on Medical Informatics; 1992 Sep 6–10; Geneva, Switzerland. Amsterdam: North-Holland; 1992. p. 1561–5.

22. *Scientific or technical report*
   Issued by funding/sponsoring agency:

   Smith P, Golladay K. Payment for durable medical equipment billed during skilled nursing facility stays. Final report. Dallas (TX): Dept. of Health and Human Services (US), Office of Evaluation and Inspections; 1994 Oct. Report No.: HHSIGOEI69200860.

   Issued by performing agency:

   Field MJ, Tranquada RE, Feasley JC, editors. Health services research: work force and educational issues. Washington: National Academy Press; 1995. Contract No.: AHCPR282942008. Sponsored by the Agency for Health Care Policy and Research.

23. *Dissertation*

   Kaplan SJ. Post-hospital home health care: the elderly's access and utilization [dissertation]. St. Louis (MO): Washington Univ.; 1995.

24. *Patent*

   Larsen CE, Trip R, Johnson CR, inventors; Novoste Corporation, assignee. Methods for procedures related to the electrophysiology of the heart. US patent 5,529,067. 1995 Jun 25.

Other Published Material

25. *Newspaper article*

   Lee G. Hospitalizations tied to ozone pollution: study estimates 50,000 admissions annually. The Washington Post 1996 Jun 21; Sect. A:3 (col. 5).

26. *Audiovisual material*

   HIV+/AIDS: the facts and the future [videocassette].
   St. Louis (MO): Mosby-Year Book; 1995.

27. *Legal material*
   Public law:

   Preventive Health Amendments of 1993, Pub. L. No. 103–183, 107 Stat. 2226 (Dec. 14, 1993).

Unenacted bill:

> Medical Records Confidentiality Act of 1995, S. 1360, 104th Cong., 1st Sess. (1995).

Code of Federal Regulations:

> Informed Consent, 42 C.F.R. Sect. 441.257 (1995).

Hearing:

> Increased Drug Abuse: the Impact on the Nation's Emergency Rooms: Hearings Before the Subcomm. on Human Resources and Intergovernmental Relations of the House Comm. on Government Operations, 103rd Cong., 1st Sess. (May 26, 1993).

28. *Map*

> North Carolina. Tuberculosis rates per 100,000 population, 1990 [demographic map]. Raleigh: North Carolina Dept. of Environment, Health, and Natural Resources, Div. of Epidemiology; 1991.

29. *Book of the Bible*

> The Holy Bible. King James version. Grand Rapids (MI): Zondervan Publishing House; 1995. Ruth 3:1–18.

30. *Dictionary and similar references*

> Stedman's Medical Dictionary. 26th ed. Baltimore: Williams & Wilkins; 1995. Apraxia; p. 119–20.

31. *Classic material*

> The Winter's Tale: act 5, scene 1, lines 13–16. The complete works of William Shakespeare. London: Rex; 1973.

Unpublished Material

32. *In press*
(Note: NLM prefers "forthcoming" because not all items will be printed.)

> Leshner AI. Molecular mechanisms of cocaine addiction. N Engl J Med. In press 1996.

Electronic Material

33. *Journal article in electronic format*

> Morse SS. Factors in the emergence of infectious diseases. Emerg Infect Dis [serial online] 1995 Jan-Mar [cited 1996 Jun 5];1(1):[24 screens]. Available from: URL: http://www.cdc.gov/ncidod/EID/eid.htm

34. *Monograph in electronic format*

> CDI, clinical dermatology illustrated [monograph on CD-ROM]. Reeves JRT, Maibach H. CMEA Multimedia Group, producers. 2nd ed. Version 2.0. San Diego: CMEA; 1995.

35. *Computer file*

> Hemodynamics III: the ups and downs of hemodynamics [computer program]. Version 2.2. Orlando (FL): Computerized Educational Systems; 1993.

Tables

Type or print out each table with double-spacing on a separate sheet of paper. Do not submit tables as photographs. Number tables consecutively in the order of their first citation in the text and supply a brief title for each. Give each column a short or abbreviated heading. Place explanatory matter in footnotes, not in the heading. Explain in footnotes all nonstandard abbreviations that are used in each table. For footnotes use the following symbols, in this sequence: *, †, ‡, §, ‖, ¶, **, ††, ‡‡, etc.

Identify statistical measures of variations, such as standard deviation and standard error of the mean.

Do not use internal horizontal and vertical rules.

Be sure that each table is cited in the text.

If you use data from another published or unpublished source, obtain permission and acknowledge them fully.

The use of too many tables in relation to the length of the text may produce difficulties in the layout of pages. Examine issues of the journal to which you plan to submit your paper to estimate how many tables can be used per 1000 words of text.

The editor, on accepting a paper, may recommend that additional tables containing important backup data too extensive to publish be deposited with an archival service, such as the National Auxiliary Publication Service in the United States, or made available by the authors. In that event an appropriate statement will be added to the text. Submit such tables for consideration with the paper.

Illustrations (Figures)

Submit the required number of complete sets of figures. Figures should be professionally drawn and photographed; freehand or typewritten lettering is unacceptable. Instead of original drawings, x-ray films, and other material, send sharp, glossy, black-and-white photographic prints, usually 127×173 mm (5×7 inches) but no larger than 203×254 mm (8×10 inches). Letters, numbers, and symbols should be clear and even throughout and of sufficient size that when reduced for publication each item will still be legible. Titles and detailed explanations belong in the legends for illustrations not on the illustrations themselves.

Each figure should have a label pasted on its back indicating the number of the figure, author's name, and top of the figure. Do not write on the back of figures or scratch or mar them by using paper clips. Do not bend figures or mount them on cardboard.

Photomicrographs should have internal scale markers. Symbols, arrows, or letters used in photomicrographs should contrast with the background.

If photographs of people are used, either the subjects must not be identifiable or their pictures must be accompanied by written permission to use the photograph (see Protection of Patients' Rights to Privacy).

Figures should be numbered consecutively according to the order in which they have been first cited in the text. If a figure has been published, acknowledge the original source and submit written permission from the copyright holder to reproduce the material.

Permission is required irrespective of authorship or publisher except for documents in the public domain.

For illustrations in color, ascertain whether the journal requires color negatives, positive transparencies, or color prints. Accompanying drawings marked to indicate the region to be reproduced may be useful to the editor. Some journals publish illustrations in color only if the author pays for the extra cost.

Legends for Illustrations

Type or print out legends for illustrations using double spacing, starting on a separate page, with Arabic numerals corresponding to the illustrations. When symbols, arrows, numbers, or letters are used to identify parts of the illustrations, identify and explain each one clearly in the legend. Explain the internal scale and identify the method of staining in photomicrographs.

Units of Measurement

Measurements of length, height, weight, and volume should be reported in metric units (meter, kilogram, or liter) or their decimal multiples.

Temperatures should be given in degrees Celsius. Blood pressures should be given in millimeters of mercury.

All hematologic and clinical chemistry measurements should be reported in the metric system in terms of the International System of Units (SI). Editors may request that alternative or non-SI units be added by the authors before publication.

Abbreviations and Symbols

Use only standard abbreviations. Avoid abbreviations in the title and abstract. The full term for which an abbreviation stands should precede its first use in the text unless it is a standard unit of measurement.

Sending the Manuscript to the Journal

Send the required number of copies of the manuscript in a heavy-paper envelope, enclosing the copies and figures in cardboard, if necessary, to prevent the photographs from being bent. Place photographs and transparencies in a separate heavy-paper envelope.

Manuscripts must be accompanied by a covering letter signed by all coauthors. This must include 1) information on prior or duplicate publication or submission elsewhere of any part of the work as defined earlier in this document; 2) a statement of financial or other relationships that might lead to a conflict of interest (see below); 3) a statement that the manuscript has been read and approved by all the authors, that the requirements for authorship as stated earlier in this document have been met, and that each author believes that the manuscript represents honest work; and 4) the name, address, and telephone number of the corresponding author, who is responsible for communicating with the other authors about revisions and final approval of the proofs. The letter should give any additional information that may be helpful to the editor, such as the type of article in the particular journal that the manuscript represents and whether the author(s) would be willing to meet the cost of reproducing color illustrations.

The manuscript must be accompanied by copies of any permissions to reproduce published material, to use illustrations or report information about identifiable people, or to name people for their contributions.

2. Separate Statements from the ICMJE

Definition of a Peer-Reviewed Journal

A peer-reviewed journal is one that has submitted most of its published articles for review by experts who are not part of the editorial staff. The number and kind of manuscripts sent for review, the number of reviewers, the reviewing procedures, and the use made of the reviewers' opinions may vary, and therefore each journal should publicly disclose its policies in its instructions to authors for the benefit of readers and potential authors.

Editorial Freedom and Integrity

Owners and editors of medical journals have a common endeavor—the publication of a reliable and readable journal, produced with due respect for the stated aims of the journal and for costs. The functions of owners and editors, however, are different. Owners have the right to appoint and dismiss editors and to make important business decisions in which editors should be involved to the fullest extent possible. Editors must have full authority for determining the editorial content of the journal. This concept of editorial freedom should be resolutely defended by editors even to the extent of their placing their positions at stake. To secure this freedom in practice, the editor should have direct access to the highest level of ownership, not only to a delegated manager.

Editors of medical journals should have a contract that clearly states the editor's rights and duties in addition to the general terms of the appointment and that defines mechanisms for resolving conflict.

An independent editorial advisory board may be useful in helping the editor establish and maintain editorial policy.

All editors and editors' organizations have the obligation to support the concept of editorial freedom and to draw major transgressions of such freedom to the attention of the international medical community.

Conflict of Interest

Conflict of interest for a given manuscript exists when a participant in the peer review and publication process—author, reviewer, and editor—has ties to activities that could inappropriately influence his or her judgment, whether or not judgment is in fact needed. Financial relationships with industry (for example, through employment, consultancies, stock ownership, honoraria, expert testimony), either directly or through immediate family, are usually considered to be the most important conflicts of interest. However, conflicts can occur for other reasons, such as personal relationships, academic competition, and intellectual passion.

Public trust in the peer review process and the credibility of published articles depend in part on how well conflict of interest is handled during writing, peer review, and editorial decision making. Bias can often be identified and eliminated by careful attention to the scientific methods and conclusions of the work. Financial relationships and their effects are less easily detected than other conflicts of interest. Participants in peer review and publication should disclose their conflicting interests, and the information should be made available so that others can judge their effects for themselves. Because readers may be less able to detect bias in review articles and editorials than in reports of original research, some journals do not accept reviews and editorials from authors with a conflict of interest.

Authors

When they submit a manuscript, whether an article or a letter, authors are responsible for recognizing and disclosing financial and other conflicts of interest that might bias their work. They should acknowledge in the manuscript all financial support for the work and other financial or personal connections to the work.

Reviewers

External peer reviewers should disclose to editors any conflicts of interest that could bias their opinions of the manuscript, and they should disqualify themselves from reviewing specific manuscripts if they believe it to be appropriate. The editors must be made aware of reviewers' conflicts of interest to interpret the reviews and judge for themselves whether the reviewer should be disqualified. Reviewers should not use knowledge of the work, before its publication, to further their own interests.

Editors and Staff

Editors who make final decisions about manuscripts should have no personal financial involvement in any of the issues they might judge. Other members of the editorial staff, if they participate in editorial decisions, should provide editors with a current description of their financial interests (as they might relate to editorial judgments) and disqualify themselves from any decisions where they have a conflict of interest. Published articles and letters should include a description of all financial support and any conflict of interest that, in the editors' judgment, readers should know about. Editorial staff should not use the information gained through working with manuscripts for private gain.

Corrections, Retractions, and "Expressions of Concern" about Research Findings

Editors must assume initially that authors are reporting work based on honest observations. Nevertheless, two types of difficulty may arise.

First, errors may be noted in published articles that require the publication of a correction or erratum of part of the work. It is conceivable that an error could be so serious as to vitiate the entire body of the work, but this is unlikely and should be handled by editors and authors on an individual basis. Such an error should not be confused with inadequacies exposed by the emergence of new scientific information in the normal course of research. The latter require no corrections or withdrawals.

The second type of difficulty is scientific fraud. If substantial doubts arise about the honesty of work, either submitted or published, it is the editor's responsibility to ensure that the question is appropriately pursued (including possible consultation with the authors). However, it is not the task of editors to conduct a full investigation or to make a determination; that responsibility lies with the institution where the work was done or with the funding agency. The editor should be promptly informed of the final decision; and if a fraudulent paper has been published, the journal must print a retraction. If this method of investigation does not result in a satisfactory conclusion, the editor may choose to publish an expression of concern with an explanation.

The retraction or expression of concern, so labeled, should appear on a numbered page in a prominent section of the journal, be listed in the contents page, and include in its heading the title of the original article. It should not simply be a letter to the editor. Ideally, the first author should be the same in the retraction as in the article, although under certain circumstances the editor may accept retractions by other responsible people. The text of the retraction should explain why the article is being retracted and include a bibliographic reference to it.

The validity of previous work by the author of a fraudulent paper cannot be assumed. Editors may ask the author's institution to assure them of the validity of earlier work published in their journals or to retract it. If this is not done they may choose to publish an announcement to the effect that the validity of previously published work is not assured.

Confidentiality

Manuscripts should be reviewed with due respect for authors' confidentiality. In submitting their manuscripts for review, authors entrust editors with the results of their scientific work and creative effort, on which their reputation and career may depend. Authors' rights may be violated by disclosure of the confidential details of the review of their manuscript. Reviewers also have rights to confidentiality, which must be respected by the editor. Confidentiality may have to be breached if dishonesty or fraud is alleged but otherwise must be honored.

Editors should not disclose information about manuscripts (including their receipt, their content, their status in the reviewing process, their criticism by reviewers, or their ultimate fate) to anyone other than the authors themselves and reviewers.

Editors should make clear to their reviewers that manuscripts sent for review are privileged communications and are the private property of the authors. Therefore, reviewers and members of the editorial staff should respect the authors' rights by not publicly discussing the authors' work or appropriating their ideas before the manuscript is published. Reviewers should not be allowed to make copies of the manuscript for their files and should be prohibited from sharing it with others, except with the permission of the editor. Editors should not keep copies of rejected manuscripts.

Opinions differ on whether reviewers should remain anonymous. Some editors require their reviewers to sign the comments returned to authors, but most either request that reviewers' comments not be signed or leave the choice to the reviewer. When comments are not signed, the reviewers' identity must not be revealed to the author or anyone else.

Some journals publish reviewers' comments with the manuscript. No such procedure should be adopted without the consent of the authors and reviewers. However, reviewers' comments may be sent to other reviewers of the same manuscript, and reviewers may be notified of the editor's decision.

Medical Journals and the Popular Media

The public's interest in news of medical research has led the popular media to compete vigorously to get information about research as soon as possible. Researchers and institutions sometimes encourage the reporting of research in the popular media before full publication in a scientific journal by holding a press conference or giving interviews.

The public is entitled to important medical information without unreasonable delay, and editors have a responsibility to play their part in this process. Doctors, however, need to have reports available in full detail before they can advise their patients about the reports' conclusions. In addition, media reports of scientific research before the work has been peer reviewed and fully published may lead to the dissemination of inaccurate or premature conclusions.

Editors may find the following recommendations useful as they seek to establish policies on these issues.

1. Editors can foster the orderly transmission of medical information from researchers, through peer-reviewed journals, to the public. This can be accomplished by an agreement with authors that they will not publicize their work while their manuscript is under consideration or awaiting publication and an agreement with the media that they will not release stories before publication in the journal, in return for which the journal will cooperate with them in preparing accurate stories (see below).

2. Very little medical research has such clear and urgently important clinical implications for the public's health that the news must be released before full publication in a journal. In such exceptional circumstances, however, appropriate authorities responsible for public health should make the decision and should be responsible for the advance dissemination of information to physicians and the media. If the author and the appropriate authorities wish to have a manuscript considered by a particular journal, the editor should be consulted before any public release. If editors accept the need for immediate release, they should waive their policies limiting prepublication publicity.

3. Policies designed to limit prepublication publicity should not apply to accounts in the media of presentations at scientific meetings or to the abstracts from these meetings (see Redundant or Duplicate Publication). Researchers who present their work at a scientific meeting should feel free to discuss their presentations with reporters, but they should be discouraged from offering more detail about their study than was presented in their talk.

4. When an article is soon to be published, editors may wish to help the media prepare accurate reports by providing news releases, answering questions, supplying advance copies of the journal, or referring reporters to the appropriate experts. This assistance should be contingent on the media's cooperation in timing their release of stories to coincide with the publication of the article.

Advertising

Most medical journals carry advertising, which generates income for their publishers, but advertising must not be allowed to influence editorial decisions. Editors must have full responsibility for advertising policy. Readers should be able to distinguish readily between advertising and editorial material. The juxtaposition of editorial and advertising material on the same products or subjects should be avoided, and advertising should not be sold on the condition that it will appear in the same issue as a particular article.

Journals should not be dominated by advertising, but editors should be careful about publishing advertisements from only one or two advertisers as readers may perceive that the editor has been influenced by these advertisers.

Journals should not carry advertisements for products that have proved to be seriously harmful to health—for example, tobacco. Editors should ensure that existing standards for advertisements are enforced or develop their own standards. Finally, editors should consider all criticisms of advertisements for publication.

Supplements

Supplements are collections of papers that deal with related issues or topics, are published as a separate issue of the journal or as a second part of a regular issue, and are usually funded by sources other than the journal's publisher. Supplements can serve useful purposes: education, exchange of research information, ease of access to focused content, and improved cooperation between academic and corporate entities. Because of the funding sources, the content of supplements can reflect biases in choice of topics and viewpoints. Editors should therefore consider the following principles.

1. The journal editor must take full responsibility for the policies, practices, and content of supplements. The journal editor must approve the appointment of any editor of the supplement and retain the authority to reject papers.

2. The sources of funding for the research, meeting, and publication should be clearly stated and prominently located in the supplement, preferably on each page. Whenever possible, funding should come from more than one sponsor.

3. Advertising in supplements should follow the same policies as those of the rest of the journal.

4. Editors should enable readers to distinguish readily between ordinary editorial pages and supplement pages.

5. Editing by the funding organization should not be permitted.

6. Journal editors and supplement editors should not accept personal favors or excessive compensation from sponsors of supplements.

7. Secondary publication in supplements should be clearly identified by the citation of the original paper. Redundant publication should be avoided.

The Role of the Correspondence Column

All biomedical journals should have a section carrying comments, questions, or criticisms about articles they have published and where the original authors can respond. Usually, but not necessarily, this may take the form of a correspondence column. The lack of such a section denies readers the possibility of responding to articles in the same journal that published the original work.

Competing Manuscripts Based on the Same Study

Editors may receive manuscripts from different authors offering competing interpretations of the same study. They have to decide whether to review competing manuscripts submitted to them more or less simultaneously by different groups or authors, or they may be asked to consider one such manuscript while a competing manuscript has been or will be submitted to another journal. Setting aside the unresolved question of ownership of data, we discuss here what editors ought to do when confronted with the submission of competing manuscripts based on the same study.

Two kinds of multiple submissions are considered: submissions by coworkers who disagree on the analysis and interpretation of their study, and submissions by coworkers who disagree on what the facts are and which data should be reported.

The following general observations may help editors and others dealing with this problem.

Differences in Analysis or Interpretation

Journals would not normally wish to publish separate articles by contending members of a research team who have differing analyses and interpretations of the data, and submission of such manuscripts should be discouraged. If coworkers cannot resolve their differences in interpretation before submitting a manuscript, they should consider submitting one manuscript containing multiple interpretations and calling their dispute to the attention of the editor so that reviewers can focus on the problem. One of the important functions of peer review is to evaluate the authors' analysis and interpretation and to suggest appropriate changes to the conclusions before publication. Alternatively, after the disputed version is published, editors may wish to consider a letter to the editor or a second manuscript from the dissenting authors. Multiple submissions present editors with a dilemma. Publication of contending manuscripts to air authors' disputes may waste journal space and confuse readers. On the other hand, if editors knowingly publish a manuscript written by only some of the collaborating team, they could be denying the rest of the team their legitimate coauthorship rights.

Differences in Reported Methods or Results

Workers sometimes differ in their opinions about what was actually done or observed and which data ought to be reported. Peer review cannot be expected to resolve this problem. Editors should decline further consideration of such multiple submissions until the problem is settled. Furthermore, if there are allegations of dishonesty or fraud, editors should inform the appropriate authorities.

The cases described above should be distinguished from instances in which independent, non-collaborating authors submit separate manuscripts based on different analyses of data that are publicly available. In this circumstance, editorial consideration of multiple submissions may be justified, and there may even be a good reason for publishing more than one manuscript because different analytical approaches may be complementary and equally valid.

I.   **Peer Review Questionnaire**

Please print.

1. Regarding the scientific manuscripts that you have peer reviewed, what are your three most common criticisms?

1	
2	
3	

2. What are the three most common mistakes that clinicians make in analyzing medical research data?

1	
2	
3	

Problematic Sections

Please circle one number for each question.	1—Introduction	2—Methods	3—Results	4—Discussion
3. Which section usually contains the most flaws?	1	2	3	4
4. Which section is most often responsible for outright rejection?	1	2	3	4
5. Which section is usually too short?	1	2	3	4
6. Which section is usually too long?	1	2	3	4

7. **What is the single most common type of flaw that results in outright rejection of a manuscript?**

   Please circle one number.

   1—Design of the study
   2—Presentation of the results
   3—Interpretation of the findings
   4—Importance of the topic

Interpretation

8. **How frequently do you encounter the following deficiencies?**

Please circle one number for each row.	Never 0%	Seldom 1%–25%	Occasionally 26%–75%	Frequently 76%–99%	Always 100%
1—Data too preliminary	0	1	2	3	4
2—Data inconclusive	0	1	2	3	4
3—Conclusions unsupported by data	0	1	2	3	4
4—Unconvincing evidence of cause and effect	0	1	2	3	4
5—Results not generalizable	0	1	2	3	4
6—Excessive bias in interpretation	0	1	2	3	4
7—Insufficient recognition of previous research	0	1	2	3	4
8—Economic consequences ignored or overinterpreted	0	1	2	3	4

9. **Of the eight problems listed above, which is most often responsible for outright rejection?**

   Enter a number from 1 to 8.

Importance of the Research

10. How frequently do you encounter the following deficiencies?

Please circle one number for each row.	Never 0%	Seldom 1%–25%	Occasionally 26%–75%	Frequently 76%–99%	Always 100%
1—Results unoriginal, predictable, or trivial	0	1	2	3	4
2—Issue outdated or no longer relevant	0	1	2	3	4
3—Results of narrow interest or highly specialized	0	1	2	3	4
4—Few or no clinical implications	0	1	2	3	4

11. Of the four problems listed above, which is most often responsible for outright rejection?

    Enter a number from 1 to 4.

Presentation

12. How frequently do you encounter the following deficiencies?

Please circle one number for each row.	Never 0%	Seldom 1%–25%	Occasionally 26%–75%	Frequently 76%–99%	Always 100%
1—Rationale confused or contradictory	0	1	2	3	4
2—Important work by others ignored	0	1	2	3	4
3—Failure to give a detailed explanation of the experimental design	0	1	2	3	4
4—Inadequate or inappropriate presentation of data	0	1	2	3	4
5—Essential data omitted or ignored	0	1	2	3	4
6—Poorly written; excessive jargon	0	1	2	3	4
7—Excessive zeal and self-promotion	0	1	2	3	4
8—Boring	0	1	2	3	4

13. Of the eight problems listed above, which is most often responsible for outright rejection?

Enter a number from 1 to 8.

14. **What are the most important lessons that you have learned about how to write and publish a medical research paper that you wish you had been taught in medical school?**

1	
2	
3	

Design

15. **How frequently do you encounter the following deficiencies?**

Please circle one number for each row.	Never 0%	Seldom 1%–25%	Occasionally 26%–75%	Frequently 76%–99%	Always 100%
1—Weak discussion	0	1	2	3	4
2—Weak conclusions	0	1	2	3	4
3—Poor presentation	0	1	2	3	4
4—Poor methods	0	1	2	3	4
5—Inadequate results	0	1	2	3	4
6—Lack of originality	0	1	2	3	4
7—Failure to adhere to journal format and policy	0	1	2	3	4
8—Inappropriate statistical analysis	0	1	2	3	4

16. **Of the eight problems listed above, which is most often responsible for outright rejection?**

 Enter a number from 1 to 8.

17. What is the single most common type of flaw that results in outright rejection of a manuscript?

18. What is the most common form of bias that leads to rejection?

19. How frequently do you encounter the following deficiencies?

Please circle one number for each row.	Never 0%	Seldom 1%–25%	Occasionally 26%–75%	Frequently 76%–99%	Always 100%
1—Inadequate control of variables	0	1	2	3	4
2—Deficiency in methodology	0	1	2	3	4
3—Research design problems	0	1	2	3	4
4—Poor conceptualization of problem or approach	0	1	2	3	4
5—Inappropriate statistical analysis	0	1	2	3	4
6—Duplication of previous work	0	1	2	3	4
7—Lack of medical supervision	0	1	2	3	4
8—Poor literature review	0	1	2	3	4
9—Inadequate protection of human subjects	0	1	2	3	4

20. Of the nine problems listed above, which is most often responsible for out-right rejection?

☐ Enter a number from 1–9.

21. Do you feel that you have adequate skills to evaluate the statistical aspects of most medical manuscripts that you are asked to review?

0—No
1—Yes

22. Which statistical techniques do you wish you knew more about?

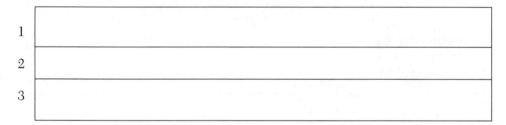

1

2

3

Statistics

23. How frequently do you encounter the following deficiencies?

Please circle one number for each row.	Never 0%	Seldom 1%–25%	Occasionally 26%–75%	Frequently 76%–99%	Always 100%
1—Insufficient information about the patient population	0	1	2	3	4
2—Inadequate sample size	0	1	2	3	4
3—Biased sample that reduced the representatives of the population studied	0	1	2	3	4
4—Confounding factors that were not taken into account	0	1	2	3	4
5—Vague end points, such as "much improved," without explanation	0	1	2	3	4
6—Straying from the hypothesis or changing the objective	0	1	2	3	4
7—Poor control of numbers (errors or inconsistences)	0	1	2	3	4

24. Of the seven problems listed above, which is the most often responsible for outright rejection?

[ ]   Enter a number from 1 to 7.

25. How frequently do you encounter the following deficiencies?

Please circle one number for each row.	Never 0%	Seldom 1%–25%	Occasionally 26%–75%	Frequently 76%–99%	Always 100%
1—Failure to collect data on variables that could influence the interpretation of results	0	1	2	3	4
2—Poor response rates in surveys	0	1	2	3	4
3—Subjects lost to follow-up or inadequate duration of follow-up in long-term studies	0	1	2	3	4
4—Extensive missing data and quality control problems	0	1	2	3	4

26. Of the four problems listed above, which is most often responsible for outright rejection?

Enter a number from 1 to 4.

Writing

27. How frequently do you encounter the following deficiencies?

Please circle one number for each row.	Never 0%	Seldom 1%–25%	Occasionally 26%–75%	Frequently 76%–99%	Always 100%
1—Poor flow of ideas	0	1	2	3	4
2—Verbiage, wordiness	0	1	2	3	4
3—Redundancy	0	1	2	3	4
4—Wrong words	0	1	2	3	4
5—Poor syntax, poor grammar	0	1	2	3	4
6—Excessive abstraction	0	1	2	3	4
7—Unnecessary complexity	0	1	2	3	4
8—Excessive compression	0	1	2	3	4
9—Unnecessary qualification	0	1	2	3	4

28. Of the nine writing problems listed above, which is most common?

Enter a number from 1 to 9.

29. When you receive a manuscript, what do you find most annoying?

Advice

30. What is your definition of a good article?

31. What advice would you give to prospective authors submitting papers to your journal?

32. Can you cite an example of what you consider the ideal paper?

33. What statistical techniques do you think will be more important in the future?

34. How could this survey have been improved?

The End

Thank you.

Reprinted by permission of Byrne Research, Ridgefield, CT.

II. Medical Journal Questionnaire

1.	What was the total paid worldwide circulation of the English language version of your journal for 1995?	
2.	What percentage of unsolicited research articles was accepted for publication in 1995?	%
3.	What was the *Science Citation Index/Journal Citation Reports* impact factor in 1995?	
4.	What is the ideal length of a manuscript for your journal (including the title page, abstract, text, references, tables, and figures)?	
Double-spaced manuscript pages:		
Pages in your journal:		
Total number of words:		
Total number of tables:		
Total number of figures:		
Total number of references:		
5.	What telephone number should potential authors use to obtain information about your journal?	
6.	What is the Web site address for your journal? http://	
7.	Is your journal stored in the Internet?	☐ No ☐ Yes
8.	What is the average turnaround time (in days) for the initial decision about acceptance?	
9.	What is the average time (in days) from submission to publication?	
10.	What percentage of the articles in your journal is peer reviewed?	%

Please add your comments on the back of this questionnaire.
Thank you.

APPENDIX C.

Sample Data Collection Form

Institute for Trauma and Emergency Care
New York Medical College

Logged __ / __ / __

ITEC

ITEC TRAUMA SYSTEMS STUDY

1. (Last name)

2. (First name)

3. (Medical record no.)

4. Age

5. Date of birth

6. Case no.

7. Sex   1 ☐ Male   2 ☐ Female

8. Admission date

9. Street

10. City

11. State

12. Zip

13. Patient arrived
    1 ☐ Directly from scene
    2 ☐ Transferred from another hospital
    3 ☐ Other

14. Hospital transferred from

16. Race   1 ☐ White   2 ☐ Black
            3 ☐ Hispanic   4 ☐ Asian   9 ☐ Other

15. Type of insurance
    1 ☐ No fault
    2 ☐ Worker's compensation
    3 ☐ Medicaid
    4 ☐ Medicare
    5 ☐ BC/BS
    6 ☐ Major Medical
    7 ☐ Self
    9 ☐ Other
    0 ☐ None

17. Location injury occurred
    1 ☐ Home   2 ☐ Travel   3 ☐ Work
    4 ☐ School   9 ☐ Other

18. Date of injury

19. Day of the week injured
    M   T   W   Th   F   Sat   Sun
    1   2   3   4   5   6   7

20. Cause of injury
    1 ☐ MVA (driver)
    2 ☐ MVA (passenger)
    3 ☐ Motorcycle
    4 ☐ ATV, 3 or 4 wheel
    5 ☐ Moped
    6 ☐ Bicycle
    7 ☐ Airplane
    8 ☐ Pedestrian hit in MVA
    9 ☐ Gunshot wound
    10 ☐ Shotgun wound
    11 ☐ Stab wound
    12 ☐ Fall
    13 ☐ Machinery
    14 ☐ Athletic
    15 ☐ Boating
    16 ☐ Assault
    17 ☐ Animal bite
    18 ☐ Human bite
    19 ☐ Other

21. Mode of arrival
    1 ☐ Private ambulance
    2 ☐ Volunteer ambulance
    3 ☐ Public ambulance
    4 ☐ Police
    5 ☐ Helicopter
    6 ☐ Fire
    7 ☐ Self
    9 ☐ Other

22. Level of care
    1 ☐ BLS   2 ☐ ALS   3 ☐ ALS & BLS
    4 ☐ Untrained   9 ☐ Other   0 ☐ None

23. Care rendered
    1 ☐ IV fluids [   ] cc   5 ☐ Immobilization
    2 ☐ MAST   6 ☐ CPR
    3 ☐ MAST not inflated   9 ☐ Other
    4 ☐ Intubation   0 ☐ None

24. Was it a suicide attempt?
    1 ☐ No   2 ☐ Yes   3 ☐ Suspected

25. If MVA, was patient wearing seat belt?
    If motorcycle, was helmet worn?
    1 ☐ No   2 ☐ Yes

26. Does patient have a history of alcohol or drug abuse?
    1 ☐ No   2 ☐ Yes
    Was patient under the influence of drugs or ETOH at injury time?
    1 ☐ No   2 ☐ Yes   3 ☐ Suspected

    BAC [   ]   Toxic screen   1 ☐ Pos   2 ☐ Neg   3 ☐ None

ADDRESS WHERE INJURY OCCURRED

27. Street	28. City	29. State
30. Cross street	31. County	32. Zip

33. Actual military time		34. Elapsed time	
a. Time of injury		a. Response time	
b. Time call was received		b. Time at scene	
c. Time of dispatch		c. Transport time	
d. Time arrived at scene		d. Time in ER	
e. Time of departure from scene		e. Time from injury to OR	
f. Time arrived at ER		f. Time from injury to 1st ER	
g. Time of triage		g. Time from injury to 2nd ER	
h. Time of departure from ER		h. Time call rec'd to OR	
i. Time arrived at 2nd ER		i. Time call rec'd to 1st ER	
j. Time arrived at OR		j. Time call rec'd to 2nd ER	
k. Time arrived at floor			

35. Trauma scoring (Value/Score)	At scene	Worst prehosp	First ER	Worst 1 hr	During transfer	Second ER
Pulse rate						
BP systolic						
Respirations per minute						
Eye opening						
Verbal response						
Motor response						
Total Glasgow score						

INITIAL HOSPITAL

36. Did patient receive	37. Units of blood
1 ☐ CAT scan of head	In first 24 hours
2 ☐ CAT scan of abdomen	
3 ☐ Swan-Ganz catheter	In first 48 hours
4 ☐ Abdominal tap	
5 ☐ Angiogram	During hospital stay
6 ☐ NMR test	
7 ☐ Intubation	

38. Prior to transfer: Procedure at transferring hospital	ICD-9
1	
2	
3	
4	
5	
6	

RECEIVING HOSPITAL

39. Did patient receive	40. Units of blood given	
1 ☐ CAT scan of head	In first 24 hours	
2 ☐ CAT scan of abdomen		
3 ☐ Swan-Ganz catheter	In first 48 hours	
4 ☐ Abdominal tap		
5 ☐ Angiogram	During hospital stay	
6 ☐ NMR test		
7 ☐ Intubation		

41. Performed in this hospital: Procedure or treatment	ICD-9
1	
2	
3	
4	
5	
6	
7	
8	

42. Complications		Day	Describe	ICD-9
☐ 0—None	1			
☐ 1—Pulmonary				
☐ 2—Cardiovascular	2			
☐ 3—Hematologic				
☐ 4—Renal	3			
☐ 5—Hepatic				
☐ 6—Infection/sepsis	4			
☐ 7—Hemorrhage				
☐ 8—Neurologic	5			
☐ 9—Other				

43. Total no. of complications		44. Days in ICU	

DISCHARGE INFORMATION

45. Final confirmed diagnosis	ICD-9	AIS/Code
1		
2		
3		
4		
5		
6		

(continued)

	ICD-9	AIS/Code
7		
8		
9		
10		

46. External cause of injury (ICD-9 E Code)

47. Date discharged   48. Disposition
                                ☐ 1—Home
49. Days in hospital   ☐ 2—Rehabilitation facility
                                ☐ 3—Other hospital
50. ISS   ☐ 4—Morgue

51.   **DIAGNOSIS RELATED GROUPS**

DRG code   DRG days allowed   Was patient an outlier?
                                              1 ☐ No   2 ☐ Yes

52. Extent of disability at discharge

INFORMATION ON DEATHS

53. Date expired   54. Time expired

55. Hours from injury to death   56. Was an autopsy performed?
                                     1 ☐ No   2 ☐ Yes

57. Where did patient die?
    1 ☐ At scene   2 ☐ In transit   3 ☐ ER   4 ☐ Hospital floor
    5 ☐ ICU   6 ☐ OR   7 ☐ Recovery room   9 ☐ Other

58. Was an organ donated from this patient?   1 ☐ No   2 ☐ Yes

59. If yes, list organs donated:

Cause of death

60. First

61. Second

62. Third

63. Fourth

64. Reviewed by (Code no.)

65. Comments:

Reprinted by permission of New York Medical College Institute for Trauma and Emergency Care, Valhalla, New York.

Medical Researcher's Directory

This appendix contains information from many fields. For journals and pharmaceutical companies in particular, it represents only a small selection of available resources. Although this directory is somewhat arbitrary, it does include top-ranking hospitals and biostatistics programs in the United States. This information was included to help you locate experts who could be valuable members of your research team.

Please do not contact these organizations or individuals to ask for free advice unless it is obvious that they want to provide it. Also, please do not use this information to sell products or services.

An asterisk (*) indicates Web sites that are of particular interest to medical researchers. Internet Web site addresses, or uniform resource locators (URLs), begin: http://.

Remember, this type of information changes rapidly, so some sites may have changed. For an updated version of this directory, visit the Williams & Wilkins home page at: http://www.wwilkins.com.

To report an error or change, please send an E-mail message to: dbyrne@snet.net.

The publisher cannot guarantee the suitability or accuracy of information, or availability of resources listed in this appendix. All information contained herein is subject to change. Mention of a specific product or company does not imply an endorsement.

Finally, to avoid frustration, remember to invest in a fast personal computer, modem, and Internet Service Provider.

Abbott Laboratories

(800) 222-6883
http://www.abbott.com

> Information on nutritional and pharmaceutical products.

Academic Press

(800) 321-5068
(800) 3131-APP
http://www.apnet.com

> Science books.

Addison Wesley Longman, Inc.

(800) 822-6339
http://www.aw.com/

> Books on statistics and computers.

Adobe Systems

(800) 833-6687
http://www.adobe.com/

> Graphic software, such as Illustrator and Persuasion.

NA = not available or not listed; Sub = subscribing information; US = United States; USN&WR = *US News & World Report*.

ADONIS

(800) 944-6415
(617) 547-8427
Fax (617) 876-7022
http://www.adonis.nl
E-mail: 7467.3144@compuserve.com

    CD-ROM article delivery service designed for medical libraries and individuals. Hundreds of scanned biomedical journals.

Agency for Health Care Policy and Research (AHCPR)

(800) 358-9295 (Publications)
(410) 381-3150
(301) 594-6662
°http://www.ahcpr.gov/

    °Clinical home page: gopher://gopher.nlm.nih.gov:70/11/hstat/ahcpr

    Information on the quality and delivery of health services.

Agency for Toxic Substances and Disease Registry

(404) 639-0500
°http://atsdr1.atsdr.cdc.gov

    Agency of the US Public Health Service. Research resources on exposure to hazardous substances.

AIDS Online Databases

See National Library of Medicine.

Airborne Express

(800) 247-2676
http://www.airborne-express.com/

    Express delivery information and tracking.

Allyn & Bacon

(800) 947-7700
Fax (515) 284-2607
Fax (515) 284-6719
http://www.abacon.com/
E-mail: ablongwood@aol.com

    Books such as Sprinthall's *Basic Statistical Analysis.*

AMA

See American Medical Association.

AMA/NET

No longer in service. See American Medical Association for new services.

Amazon.com Books

(800) 201-7575
http://www.amazon.com/

    Large online bookstore.

America Online

(800) 827-6364
http://www.aol.com

    Internet Online services.

American Academy of Arts and Sciences

(617) 576-5000
Fax (617) 576-5050
http://www.amacad.org

    Honorary society. Publications include *Daedalus.*

American Association for the Advancement of Science (AAAS)

(202) 326-6400
Membership (202) 326-6417
Fax (202) 371-9526
Fax (202) 289-4021
http://www.aaas.org/

    135,000 members. The journal *Science* and information on science and AAAS membership.

American Board of Family Practice

(606) 269-5626
http://www.abfp.org

    Journal.

American Cancer Society

(404) 329-7554 (Research)
Fax (404) 321-4669
http://www.cancer.org
E-mail: dwillis@cancer.org

    Cancer news and applications for research grants.

American Clinical and Climatological Association

(507) 284-3320

    Association of internists with an interest in clinical research.

American College of Epidemiology

(301) 251-0594
http://amcollepi.org/ace/ace.htm

The journal *Annals of Epidemiology* and a newsletter.

American College of Physicians

(800) 523-1546 ext. 2600
http://www.acponline.org/

Books, such as Hall's *How to Write a Paper*, and information on internal medicine.

American College of Preventive Medicine (ACPM)

(202) 466-2044
Fax (202) 466-2662
http://www.cais.net/acpm/

National organization of 2000 physicians involved in disease prevention.

American Family Physician

(202) 687-1631
(800) 274-2237
Editor (816) 333-9700
http://www.aafp.org
http://www.aafp.org/family/afp/
http://www.aafp.org/familymed

Journal for physicians who specialize in family practice, general practice, or internal medicine.

American Federation for Medical Research (AFCR)

(609) 848-7072
(609) 848-1000
(202) 429-5161
Fax (202) 223-4579
http://www.afmr.org
http://www.afcr.org/
E-mail: afmr@sba.com

11,000 members who are clinical scientists younger than 43 years old. Formerly the American Federation for Clinical Research. *AFCR Newsletter.*

American Health Consultants, Inc.

(800) 688-2421
(404) 262-7436
http://www.ahcpub.com/

Medical economics company.

American Home Products

(201) 660-5000
http://www.ahp.com

Information on pharmaceuticals, biotechnology, and medical devices.

American Journal of Clinical Pathology

(312) 738-1336 ext. 314
http://www.ascp.org

American Journal of Nursing Company

(212) 582-8820
Sub (800) 627-0484
Sub (303) 604-1464
Books (800) 962-6651 ext. 6700
http://www.ajn.org/

Lippincott's nursing center. Educational material and books, such as Polit-O'Hara's *Nursing Research.*

American Journal of Obstetrics and Gynecology

(614) 486-4044
(800) 325-4177 ext. 4591
Fax (614) 846-6176
http://www.mosby.com/mosby/periodicals/medical/ajog/ob.html

American Journal of Ophthalmology

(310) 825-8587
http://www.ajo.com/

American Journal of Physical Medicine and Rehabilitation

(317) 845-4200
Fax (317) 845-4299
http://www.wwilkins.com
E-mail: aap@indy.net

American Journal of Psychiatry

Editor (202) 682-6020
Fax (202) 682-6016
http://www.appi.org/aip/ajptoc.html

Up-to-date information for authors and other advice.

American Marketing Association

(800) 262-1150
(312) 648-0536
http://www.ama.org/

NTC Handbook for Customer Satisfaction.

American Mathematical Society

(800) 321-4267
(401) 455-4000
Fax (401) 331-3842
http://www.ams.org/
http://e-math.ams.org/
E-mail: ams@ams.org

> 30,000 members. Membership information, advanced mathematical books, and related resources.

American Medical Association (AMA)

(800) 621-8335
(312) 645-5000
(312) 464-5000
Answer center (312) 464-4818
Member service system (800) 262-3211
Fax on request service (800) 621-8335
°http://www.ama-assn.org/

> *JAMA* and other journals as well as many services, including a database for finding a specific physician in the US, catalog of books and gifts, and ICD and CPT coding books.

American Medical Informatics Association (AMIA)

(301) 657-1291
Fax (301) 657-1296
http://amia2.amia.org/
http://www.amia.org
E-mail: mail@amia2.amia.org

> Meeting and publication information regarding medical information systems.

American Medical News

(312) 464-5000
http://www.ama-assn.org/public/journals/am-news/amnews.htm

> Online version of the American Medical Association's weekly newspaper.

American Medical Publishers Association (AMPA)

(516) 423-0075

> *AMPA Newsletter.*

American Medical Student Association (AMSA) Foundation

(703) 620-6600 ext. 202
http://www.amsa.org/

News about national and local chapters. Information on their publication *The New Physician.*

American Medical Writers Association (AMWA)

(301) 493-0003
Fax (301) 493-6384
http://www.amwa.org.amwa
E-mail: amwa@amwa.org

> *AMWA Journal* and services for professional communicators in the biomedical sciences. Freelance or full-time medical writers or editors.

American Pharmaceutical Research Companies

(800) 862-5110
http://www.phrma.org

> Drug information from a group of 100 pharmaceutical companies.

American Physiological Society (APS)

(301) 530-7164
Fax (301) 571-8313
http://www.faseb.org/aps
http://oac.hsc.uth.tmc.edu/apstracts/
E-mail: info@aps.faseb.org

> Online abstracts of APS publications, sometimes 4 months before publication.

American Psychiatric Association

(202) 682-6000
http://www.psych.org
http://www.appi.org

> Policy, news, and publication information. Catalog of American Psychiatric Press, Inc. books and CD-ROMs.

American Psychological Association (APA)

(800) 374-2721
(202) 336-5500
http://www.apa.org
E-mail:webmaster@apa.org

> Information and publications, such as the *Publication Manual of the American Psychological Association.*

American Public Health Association

(202) 789-5600
http://www.apha.org/

> News, conferences, and publications.

American Society for Clinical Investigation (ASCI)

(800) 257-8290
(609) 848-1000
http://mmg.im-med.umich.edu.edu/asci/

2400 medical researchers. *Journal of Clinical Investigation.*

American Society of Health-System Pharmacists

(301) 657-3000
http://www.ashp.org

Educational material for hospital pharmacists.

American Statistical Association

(703) 684-1221
Fax (703) 684-2037
http://www.amstat.org/
E-mail: asainfo@amstat.org

18,390 members. Statistical resources and publications.

Amgen, Inc.

(800) 282-6436
(805) 447-1000
Fax (805) 447-1010
http://www.amgen.bio.com http://wwwext.amgen.com/cgi-bin/genobject

Global biotechnology company. Discovers, develops, manufactures, and markets human therapeutics based on advanced cellular and molecular biology.

Andersen Consulting

(212) 708-4400
http://www.ac.com/

Andersen's Healthcare Industry Group specializes in the medical field.

Annals of Internal Medicine

(215) 351-2400
(215) 351-2628
Sub (800) 523-1546 ext. 2600
Fax (215) 351-2644
http://www.acponline.org

Journal published by the American College of Physicians.

AnyBook International (formerly BookServe International)

(800) 888-8139
http://www.anybook.com/
E-mail: anybook@anybook.com

Online bookstore.

AORN Online

http://www.aorn.org/

Service of the Association of Operating Room Nurses, Inc.

APM Management Consultants

(312) 470-8600

Medical consulting firm.

Apple Computer, Inc.

(408) 996-1010
http://www.apple.com

Resources for Apple computer users.

Appleton & Lange

(800) 451-3794
(800) 423-1359
(203) 406-4500
http://www.appleton-lange.com

Medical books, such as Dawson-Saunders' *Basic and Clinical Biostatistics.*

Archives of General Psychiatry

(312) 464-5000
(800) AMA-2350
(312) 670-7827
Editorial office (212) 746-3771
Fax (312) 464-5831
http://www.ama-assn.org/
E-mail: archives-comments@ama-assn.org

Journal.

Archives of Internal Medicine

Sub (312) 464-5000
Editorial office (520) 326-8334
Fax (520) 326-6188
http://www.ama-assn.org/

Journal.

Archives of Surgery

(800) 262-2350
(312) 670-7827
Editorial office (510) 437-4965
http://www.ama-assn.org

Journal.

Aries Systems Corporation

(508) 975-7570
Fax (508) 975-3811
http://www.ariessys.com/
E-mail: webmaster@ariessys.com

Knowledge Finder electronic literature
searching system, CD-ROMs, and searching
software.

Aspen Publishers, Inc.

(800) 638-8437
(301) 417-7500
Fax (301) 417-7650
°http://www.aspenpub.com

Books on managed care and other health
care topics, such as Morton's *A Study Guide
to Epidemiology and Biostatistics*. Directory
of useful Web sites (AspenLINK).

Association of Medical Illustrators (AMI)

(404) 350-7900
Fax (404) 351-3348
http://medical-illustrators.org/

Organization of 1000 graphic artists who
specialize in medical applications. *Journal of
Biocommunications*, a newsletter, and the
AMI source book (with examples of members' work).

Association of Teachers of Technical Writing

(407) 823-2212
http://english.ttu.edu/ATTW/

Technical Communication Quarterly.

AT&T Labs Research

(800) 400-1447
Lucent Technologies (888) 4-LUCENT
Internet access (800) 967-5363
E-mail access (800) 242-6005
http://www.research.att.com/
http://www.lucent.com

Information on computers and communication technology.

AT&T Toll-Free Internet Directory

(800) 555-1212
http://www.tollfree.att.net/dir800/

Toll-free numbers listed with AT&T.

Avicenna

(800) AVICENNA
http://www.avicenna.com

MEDLINE access and other resources for
physicians.

Barnes & Noble

(800) 668-7053
http://www.barnesandnoble.com

Online bookstore.

Barnes-Jewish Hospital

(314) 362-5000
http://mcfsun1.wustl.edu/medcenter/

Hospital ranked #12 in 1997 by US News
& World Report.

Bayer Corporation

(412) 394-5500
(800) 662-2927
(412) 777-2000
http://www.bayer.com

Pharmaceutical company.

Biosciences Information Services (BIOSIS)

(215) 569-4800
(800) 523-4806
(215) 587-4847
Fax (215) 587-2016
http://www.biosis.org

Nonprofit organization. Access to abstracts
in the life sciences.

Biosoft

(314) 524-8029
http://www.biosoft.com

Scientific software, including RefSys and
AutoBiblio reference management software.

BMDP Statistical Software, Inc.

See SPSS.

Boehringer Ingelheim Corporation

(203) 798-9988

http://www.boehringer-ingelheim.com

Pharmaceutical research information.

Book Garden Gallery

http://www.bookgarden.com
Online bookstore.

BookServe International.

See AnyBook International.

Brain Surgery Information Center

Fax (212) 879-2995
°http://www.brain-surgery.com
E-mail: jrmbrain@aol.com

Nontechnical information on brain surgery
from John R. Mangiardi, MD, Chief of Neu-
rosurgery at Lenox Hill Hospital in New
York City.

Brigham and Women's Hospital

(617) 732-5500
Fax (617) 732-4144
http://gopher.bwh.harvard.edu/

Hospital ranked #9 in 1997 by USN&WR.
Affiliated with Harvard Medical School.

Bristol-Myers Squibb

(800) 648-2694
(609) 897-2000
http://www.bms.com/squibb/toc.html

Pharmaceutical information.

**British Library Document Supply Centre
(BLDSC)**

+44-1937-546060
Fax +44-1937-546333
http://www.bl.uk/dsc/

Document delivery service and other information.

British Medical Journal

+44(0)171-387-4499
Fax +44(0)171-383-6418
°http://www.bmj.com/bmj/
E-mail: 100730.1250@compuserve.com

Detailed information for authors, a catalog
of medical books, and full-text and archived
articles.

**BRS/COLLEAGUE and BRS Information
Technologies**

See Ovid Technologies, Inc.

Bulletin Board for Libraries (BUBL)

http://bubl.ac.uk/

British library information for the academic
and research community.

Bureau of the Census

See US Census Bureau.

Byrne Research

(203) 431-4184
Fax (203) 438-9544
E-mail: dbyrne@snet.net

The author's consulting firm.

California Institute of Technology

(818) 395-6811
http://www.caltech.edu
http://www.ama.caltech.edu (Applied Mathematics)

Mathematical resources.

Cambridge Scientific Abstracts

(800) 843-7751
(301) 951-1400
°http://www.csa.com

Literature searching and Internet database
service.

Cambridge University Press

(800) 221-4512
Book orders (800) 872-7423
http://www.cup.cam.ac.uk/

Books such as Huth's *Scientific Style and
Format: The CBE Manual for Authors, Editors and Publishers.*

Canadian Medical Association Journal

(800) 663-7336 ext. 2307
(613) 731-8610 ext. 2307
http://www.cma.ca/journals/cmaj/
E-mail: pubs@cma.ca

Carl Corporation

See UnCover Company–Carl Corporation.

Carnegie Mellon University

(412) 268-2000
Department of Statistics (412) 268-8725
°http://lib.stat.cmu.edu
°http://lib.stat.cmu.edu/otherplaces/

> Statistical resource. List of other helpful sites and links to statistical departments around the world.

Cartoon Bank

(800) 897-8666
(914) 478-5527
Fax (914) 478-5604
http://www.cartoonbank.com

> Database of cartoons. For a fee, searches any topic and provides cartoons for slide presentations or publications.

CASDDS

(800) 678-4337
°http://info.cas.org/

> Chemical abstract service and document detective service.

CCC (Copyright Clearance Center, Inc.)

(508) 750-8400
Fax (508) 750-4470
http://www.copyright.com/

CDC

See Centers for Disease Control and Prevention.

CDP Colleague

See Ovid Technologies, Inc.

Cell

(617) 661-7057
Fax (617) 661-7061
°http://www.cell.com/
E-mail: editor@cell.com

> Journal.

Centers for Disease Control and Prevention (CDC)

(404) 639-3311
(404) 332-4569
(404) 639-0849
(404) 728-0545

(770) 469-4098
Fax (770) 469-0681
Office of Public Affairs (public inquiries and publications) (404) 639-3534
Job hotline (404) 332-4577
°http://www.cdc.gov/
http://www.cdc.gov/travel/travel.html
http://wonder.cdc.gov
http://www.cdc.gov/epo/epi/epiinfo.htm

> Easy-to-use and inexpensive software for public health work (e.g., database, word processing, statistics). CDC WONDER provides access to information about the CDC and access to many publications.

CenterWatch, Inc.

(617) 247-2327
Fax (617) 247-2535
http://www.centerwatch.com
E-mail: cntrwatch@aol.com

> Clinical trials listing service.

Central Society for Clinical Research (CSCR)

(312) 951-5610

> 1294 medical research experts. *Journal of Laboratory and Clinical Medicine.*

Chemical Abstracts Service (CAS)

(614) 447-3711
http://info.cas.org/

> One of the world's largest and most comprehensive databases of chemical information. The primary databases, Chemical Abstracts and Registry, include 13 million abstracts of chemistry-related and patent literature and more than 16 million substance records.

Cleveland Clinic Hospital

(216) 444-2200
Foundation (216) 444-8950
Fax (216) 444-5446
http://www.ccf.org/CCFMain.html

> Hospital ranked #6 in 1997 by USN&WR. Research and education resources.

Clinical Orthopaedics and Related Research

Sub (800) 638-3030
http://www.lrpub.com/sites/corr/

> Orthopaedic journal.

Clinical Trials Posting

http://www.clinicaltrials.com

Patient registry and information about clinical trials.

CliniWeb

http://www.ohsu.edu/cliniweb/

Service from the Oregon Health Sciences University. Provides clinical health information categorized by medical subject heading (MeSH) terms.

Columbia/HCA Healthcare

(800) COLUMBIA
http://www.columbia.net/

Large health care services provider. Online resources.

Columbia Presbyterian Medical Center

(212) 854-1754
(212) 305-2500
Department of Medical Informatics
   (212) 305-5780
Department of Statistics (212) 854-3652
Division of Biostatistics (212) 305-9398
Mathematics Department (212) 854-4112
http://cpmcnet.columbia.edu/health.sci/
http://www.cpmc.columbia.edu/
http://www.columbia.edu/cu/healthwise
http://www.stat.columbia.edu/index.html
http://cpmcnet.columbia.edu/dept/sph/biostat/
http://www.math.columbia.edu/

Resources for medical researchers, including Healthwise, a health education and wellness program. Hospital ranked # 16 in 1997 by USN&WR.

Commonwealth Scientific and Industrial Research Organizations (CSIRO)

(06) 276-6766
Fax (06) 276-6766
http://www.csiro.au/

Scientific research agency of the Australian government.

Community of Science Web Server

http://cos.gdb.org/

Consortium of research institutions. Scientific expertise, funding information, and MEDLINE access.

Compaq

(800) 888-5858
(713) 370-0670
DirectPlus (800) 888-4431
Dealer locator (800) 231-0900
http://www.compaq.com/

Personal computers.

Comprehensive Epidemiologic Data Resource

(301) 903-4674
http://cedr.lbl.gov

Epidemiologic data about energy facilities. Public access to radiation exposure and outcome databases.

CompuServe

(800) 848-8199
(800) 848-8990
(800) 858-8199
(800) 336-6823
http://www.compuserve.com/

Medical and other online services. Access to databases, such as PaperChase.

Computerworld

(508) 879-0700
Sub (800) 669-1002
Fax (508) 820-8129
http://www.computerworld.com

Weekly computer journal of computer developments. Up-to-date online information.

Conceptual Software, Inc.

(800) 328-2686
(713) 721-4200
Fax (713) 721-4298
http://www.conceptual.com/

DBMS/COPY data conversion software and Data Muncher software.

Congressional Information Service, Inc. (CIS)

(800) 227-2477
(800) 638-8380
(301) 654-1550
http://www.cispubs.com

Access to US government information.

Consultant

(203) 661-0600

    Journal.

Contemporary Surgery

(310) 376-8788
Fax (310) 376-9043

    Journal.

Cool Medical Site of the Week

http://www.maxface.com/~wcd/cmsotw.html
http://www.hooked.net/users/wcd/cmsotw.html

    Links to entertaining medical Web sites. Try
the previous cool medical sites listed.

Copy Editor

(212) 995-0112
Fax (212) 995-2147
http://www.copyeditor.com

    National newsletter for professional copy
editors.

Corel WordPerfect

(800) 205-4295
Technical support (800) 321-5906
http://www.wordperfect.com/
http://wp.novell.com

    Popular WordPerfect word processing soft-
ware. Information on other products and
services, including Grammatik grammar-
checking software.

Cornell University

(607) 254-INFO
(607) 255-2000
Statistics Center (607) 255-8066
http://www.cornell.edu
http://www.med.cornell.edu/
http://www.stat.cornell.edu

    Graduate school ranked #4 in mathematical
statistics in 1996 by USN&WR.

Council of Biology Editors, Inc.

(847) 480-6349
(847) 480-9080
Fax (847) 480-9282
http://www.edoc.com/cbe/
E-mail: cbehdqts@aol.com

Organization for people interested in improving communication in the life sciences.
CBE Views.

Critical Care Nurse

(800) 345-8112
(714) 362-2000 ext. 532
http://www.iqnow.com/access/join.html

    *Journal of the American Association of Crit-
ical Care Nurses.*

**Cumulative Index to Nursing and Allied
Health Literature (CINAHL)**

(818) 409-8005
(800) 959-7167
http://www.cinahl.com

    Print, CD-ROM, and online databases.

Current Contents

See Institute for Scientific Information, Inc.

Cytel Software Corporation

(617) 661-2011
http://www.cytel.com/

    StatXact nonparametric-test software and
Egret and Egret SIZ software.

DataEase International

(800) 243-5123
Sales (203) 374-8000
Technical support (203) 374-2825
http://www.multi-ware.com/dataease.html

    Easy-to-use database management software.

Data Muncher

See Conceptual Software, Inc.

DataStar

See Knight-Ridder Information, Inc.

Declaration of Helsinki

http://www.sar.co.uk/helsinki.htm

    Recommendations for medical physicians
performing biomedical research involving
human subjects.

Delphi

(800) 695-4005
http://www.delphi.com

Online information services. Information on special interest groups and forums.

U.S. Department of Health and Human Services

(202) 619-0257
http://www.os.dhhs.gov/

Programs and services to locate the appropriate agency or publication for research problems.

DIALOG Information Services, Inc.

See Knight-Ridder Information, Inc.

DialogLink

See Knight-Ridder Information, Inc.

DIMDI (German Institute for Medical Documentation and Information)

+(49)-221-4724-1
http://www.dimdi.de

German-based health database service.

Dms4Cite

(201) 666-6262

Bibliographic database software.

Doctor's Guide to the Internet

°http://www.pslgroup.com/docguide.htm

Latest medical literature at a glance. Resources and information on conferences and new drugs.

Doctors of the World

(888) 817-4357
(212) 529-1556
(212) 226-9890
Fax (212) 226-7026
http://www.igc.apc.org/ia/mb/dow.html
E-mail: DOW@igc.apc.org

Organization that provides medical care and expertise to people around the world who cannot afford to pay.

Doody Publishing's Health Sciences Book Reviews

(800) 219-9500
http://www1.doody.com/web/dej.htm

Reviews of medical books.

Duke University Hospital

(919) 684-8111
Institute of Statistics and Decision Sciences
(919) 684-8029
Fax (919) 681-8921
http://www.mc.duke.edu/depts/som/
http://www.mc.duke.edu/
http://www.isds.duke.edu

Hospital ranked #4 in 1997 by USN&WR.

Eastern Paralyzed Veterans Association

(718) 803-EPVA
(800) 795-3620
Fax (718) 803-0414
°http://www.epva.org

Spinal cord injury research, programs, and publications.

EBSCO Publishing

(800) 653-2726
(508) 356-6500
Fax (508) 356-5640
°http://www.epnet.com
E-mail: ep@epnet.com

Electronic MEDLINE and CINAHL (nursing) databases, CD-ROM software, and a searching interface.

Editorial Eye

(703) 683-0683
Fax (703) 683-4915
http://www.eeicom.com/eye/

12-page monthly newsletter for writers, editors, designers, project managers, and communication specialists.

Egret SIZ.

See Cytel Software (617) 661-2011.

Power and sample size software.

Electronic Media Documentation and Online Concepts (EMDOC)

(516) 997-0699
(800) 282-2720
http://www.csa.com/emdocsde.html

EMBASE Document delivery service. Use Dialog to perform a search.

Elements of Style

http://www.cc.columbia.edu/acis/bartleby/strunk

Online version of the classic writing book.

Eli Lilly and Company

(317) 276-2000
(800) 545-5979
http://www.lilly.com/

Pharmaceutical information and career opportunities.

Elsevier Publishing Company

(212) 989-5800
(914) 524-9200
(888) 437-4636
http://www.elsevier.nl/

Medical books and journals.

Emergency Medicine

(800) 976-4040
http://www.emedmag.com

Journal.

EndNote

See Niles & Associates, Inc.

Entrez Document Retrieval System

(301) 496-2475
°http://www.ncbi.nlm.nih.gov/entrez

Literature searches of the molecular biology
subset of MEDLINE. Genetic sequence
searching. Access through National Center
for Biotechnology Information.

Environmental Protection Agency

(202) 260-2090
°http://www.epa.gov/

Resources on air and water quality, pollution, and pesticides.

Epi Info, USD, Inc.

(770) 469-4098
Tech info (404) 728-0545
Fax (770) 469-0681
http://www.usd-inc.com

Easy-to-use and inexpensive software.

European Association of Science Editors

71 3889668
Fax 71 3833092
http://www.compulink.co.uk/~ease-eurscieditors/
E-mail: ease_moc@cix.compulink.co.uk

European Science Editing.

European Medical Writers Association

http://www.netlink.co.uk/users/emwa/index.html
E-mail: marian@molesoft.demon.co.uk

Newsletter, annual conference, and refer-
rals.

Evidence Based Medicine

http://hiru.mcmaster.ca/ebm/
http://www.acponline.org/journals/ebm/ebm-
menu.htm
http://cebm.jr2.ox.ac.uk/

Excerpta Medica

(212) 916-1161
(908) 874-8550
http://www.excerptamedica.com/home3.html

Medical communications group.

Excel

See Microsoft

ExperNet

(800) 266-2865
Fax (805) 298-4388
http://www.expernet.com

Telephone advice from independent information technology consultants for a fee.

Faxon

(800) 766-0039
(617) 329-3350
http://www.faxon.com/

Serial publication subscription agency.

FDA

See Food and Drug Administration.

**Federal Emergency Management Agency
(FEMA)**

(202) 646-4600
http://www.fema.gov/

Information on disasters.

Federal Express

(800) 463-3339
http://www.fedex.com

Online service, tracking, and software.

Federal Web Locator

http://www.law.vill.edu/fed-agency/fedwebloc.html

Provided by the Villanova Center for Information Law and Policy. Tool for finding the Internet sites of federal agencies.

Food and Drug Administration (FDA)

(800) 638-2041
(301) 443-1970
(301) 443-2410
Office of Consumer Affairs (301) 443-1594
°http://www.fda.gov

Information about the safety of food, drugs, and devices, including drug approval information, news releases, and important alerts.

Ford Foundation

(212) 573-5000
http://www.fordfound.org/

Grant information.

Foundation for Advances in Medicine and Science

(201) 818-1010
Fax (201) 818-0086
http://www.scanning-fams.org/

Scanning: The Journal of Scanning Microscopies.

Foundation Center

(800) 424-9836
(212) 620-4230
http://fdncenter.org/

Grant information.

Galaxy

http://doradus.einet.net/galaxy.html

Tool for searching the Internet.

Gartner Group, Inc.

(203) 964-0096
http://www.gartner.com/

E-mail: info@gartner.com

Information technology consultants.

Genie

(800) 638-9636
http://www.GEnie.com

Online computer service. Text-based searching. Monthly fee and charge for searching databases.

Genome Database

(410) 955-9705
http://gdbwww.gdb.org
E-mail: help@gdb.org

International collaboration in support of the human genome project.

Genuine Article

(215) 386-0100 ext. 1140
(215) 386-4399
Fax (215) 386-4343
http://www.isinet.com/

Full-text document delivery service from the Institute for Scientific Information, Inc.

Getty (J. Paul) Trust

(310) 393-4244
http://www.getty.edu/getty.html

Grant information.

GlaxoWellcome, Inc.

(919) 248-2100
http://www.glaxowellcome.co.uk/

Information on pharmaceuticals.

Glen McPherson's Essential Book List

http://www.stat.wisc.edu/statistics/consult/stat-book.html

Recommended statistical books.

Glencoe Division of McGraw-Hill

(800) 848-1567
(800) 334-7344
Fax (614) 860-1877
http://www.glencoe.com

Books such as Sabin's *Gregg Reference Manual.*

GLIM (Generalised Linear Interactive Modelling)

http://www.nag.co.uk/1h/stats/GDGE

Global Health Network

(412) 624-5408
http://www.pitt.edu/HOME/GHNet/
E-mail: amy+@pitt.edu

> Alliance of experts working toward disease prevention.

Grammatik

See Corel WordPerfect.

Grateful Med

See National Library of Medicine.

Harvard University Medical School

(617) 432-1000
(617) 432-1171
School of Public Health, Department of Biostatistics (617) 432-1056
Fax (617) 739-1781
Countway Library of Medicine (617) 432-4888
Department of Statistics (617) 495-5497
(617) 495-2170
°http://www.med.harvard.edu
http://biosun1.harvard.edu/
http://www.med.harvard.edu/countway/
http://www.fas.harvard.edu/~stats/
http://www.math.harvard.edu/

Hayes Microcomputer Products, Inc.

(770) 840-9200
Facts on demand (800) 429-3739
http://www.hayes.com/

> Information on modems.

Health Care Financing Administration (HCFA)

(410) 786-3000
http://www.hcfa.gov

> Health hotlines. Information on Medicare, Medicaid, and DRGs.

Health Care Information Resources

http://www-hsl.mcmaster.ca/tomflem/top.html

> Internet resources from Canada.

Healthcare Computing Publications, Inc.

(718) 499-5910
http://www.healthcarecomputing.com

> Newsletter with medical software reviews.

HealthGate

(800) 434-4283
°http://www.healthgate.com
E-mail: info@healthgate.com

> Access to MEDLINE and other health databases.

Health and Human Services (Department of)

See Department of Health and Human Services.

HealthNet

(613) 990-3305
http://debra.dgbt.doc.ca/~mike/home.html
E-mail: mike@debra.dgbt.doc.ca

> Canadian health care information demonstration project.

Health Resource, Inc.

(800) 949-0090
(501) 329-5272
Fax (501) 329-9489
°http://www.thehealthresource.com

> One of the first medical information services in the US. In-depth, individualized reports and searches of the international literature for physicians, health care professionals, and patients provided for a fee.

Health Resources and Services Administration

(301) 443-2216
(301) 443-6707
http://www.os.dhhs.gov/hrsa/

> Division of the Department of Health and Human Services. Provides resources and information for medically needy populations.

HealthSeek

°http://www.healthseek.com
http://www.healthseek.com/reseprog.htm
E-mail: fisher@healthseek.com

> Good place to start looking for information on the Internet because it has many helpful links, grouped by specialty.

Health Services Research

(202) 223-2477
Sub (708) 450-9952
Fax (202) 835-8972

http://www.xnet.com/~hret/AHSR

Journal.

Healthtouch

http://www.healthtouch.com

Information on drugs, side effects, and other health topics.

HealthWorld Online

http://www.healthy.net
E-mail: hwinfo@healthy.net

Information on health food, holistic health products, and self-managed care. MEDLINE access.

Healthy Concepts

(914) 638-1619

Program planning, research, and evaluation consulting services.

Healthy People 2000 Report

See US Government Printing Office.

Hewlett-Packard

Technical line/direct ordering (800) 538-8787
Support with current products (208) 323-2551
Automated support access (800) 333-1917
Technical support billed to your telephone number (900) 555-1500
Part numbers (916) 783-0804
Parts and manuals (800) 227-8164
http://www.hp.com

Laser printers, fax machines, personal computers, and other electronic equipment. Technical information and answers to frequently asked questions.

Hospital Medicine

(908) 874-8550
http://www.elsevier.com

Illustrated review of clinical medicine for primary care physicians.

Hospital Physician: Internal and Family Medicine Edition

(610) 975-4541

Journal.

Hospital Practice

(612) 832-7889
(612) 835-3222
http://www.mcgraw-hill.com/legal-medical-pros/hospract.htm

Journal.

Hospital of the University of Pennsylvania

(215) 662-4000
http://www.med.upenn.edu/

Hospital ranked #14 in 1997 by USN&WR.

HospitalWeb

http://neuro-www.mgh.harvard.edu/hospital-web.nclk

Links to hospitals around the world.

Houghton Mifflin Company

(800) 225-3362
Fax (800) 634-7568
http://www.hmco.com/trade/

Books, such as the *American Heritage Dictionary of the English Language*.

Howard Hughes Medical Institute

(301) 215-8889
Fax (301) 215-8888
http://www.hhmi.org

Research grants.

Humane Medicine

(613) 731-9331
http://www.cup.org

Journal published by Cambridge University Press.

HyperDOC

(800) 272-4787
http://www.nlm.nih.gov/

News from the National Library of Medicine.

IBM

(800) 426-3333
(520) 574-4600
Lotus/Desktop Products
(508) 988-2500
http://www.ibm.com/
http://www.software.ibm.com/
http://www.lotus.com

Computer and software information, such as Lotus and Freelance Graphics.

IHP Net Health Resources

°http://www.interaccess.com/ihpnet/health.html

List of links to other health-related sites.

Index Medicus

(202) 512-1800
http://kumchttp.mc.ukans.edu/service/dykes/TIP SHEET/indxmed.html

See National Library of Medicine.

Information Access Company

(800) 227-8431
Fax (415) 378-5369
http://www.iacnet.com

Full text for more than 100 journals, such as *JAMA*, health references, and CD-ROMs.

Inforonics, Inc.

(508) 486-8976
http://www.titlenet.com

Services for the publishing industry.

Institute of Mathematical Statistics (IMS)

(510) 783-8141
Fax (510) 783-4131
http://www.stat.ucla.edu/ims/
E-mail: ims@stat.berkeley.edu

4000 members. *IMS Bulletin* and links to other statistical sites.

Institute of Medicine (IOM)

(202) 334-2169
Fax (202) 334-1694
http://www2.nas.edu/iom/

1024 members. Part of the National Academy of Sciences. Scientific health information.

Institute for Safe Medication Practices

(215) 956-9181
(215) 947-7566
http://www.geohealthweb.com/ISMP/

Drug interaction information.

Institute for Scientific Information, Inc.

(215) 386-0100
(800) 336-4474
(800) 523-1850
°http://www.isinet.com

Current Contents, Science Citation Index, literature searching products, chemical databases, and impact factors on CD-ROM and other media.

Insurance Institute for Highway Safety

(703) 247-1500
Fax (703) 247-1678
°http://www.hwysafety.org

Free subscriptions to the newsletter *Status Report.* Information on motor vehicle crashes, trauma, and prevention.

Interactive Medical Student Lounge

http://falcon.cc.ukans.edu/~nsween/
E-mail: nsween@falcon.cc.ukans.edu

Links and resources for medical and pre-medical students.

International Biometric Society (IBS)

(202) 223-9669
Fax (202) 223-9569
Eastern North American Region
(703) 437-4377
(703) 525-1191
Western North American Region
(307) 766-3341
http://www.stats.gla.ac.uk/~adrian/biometrics/biometric.html
E-mail: 75703.1407@compuserve.com

6500 members. Statistical information and resources.

International Committee of Medical Journal Editors

(215) 351-2660
http://www.acponline.org/journals/resource/unifreqr.htm

Uniform Requirements for Manuscripts Submitted to Biomedical Journals.

International Conference on Harmonisation

http://amherst.edu/amherst/admin/library/amherstGPO.html

http://members.aol.com/Natalie415/index.html
http://hkusuc.hku.hk/ctc/htext301.htm
http://hkusuc.hku.hk/ctc/est.htm
http://cos/gdb/org/repos/fr/toc/960717.html

Guidelines on the structure and content of clinical study reports. See Federal Register 1996;61:37319–37343.

International Medical Communications

(502) 456-1099
Fax (502) 456-1080
°http://www.inmed.com

Editing and writing, statistical analysis, medical illustration, marketing, and other medical communication services.

International Medicine and Health Network

(804) 828-2905
http://griffin/vcu.edu/html.biomedelinmednet.html

CommonHealthNet, run by an international consortium. Global telemedicine and health care telecommunications services.

International Society for Clinical Biostatistics (ISCB)

+45 48 48 4100
http://ourworld.compuserve.com/homepages/David_W_Warne/

Clinical research statistics and methodology.

International Statistical Institute

+31 70 3375737
http://www.cbs.nl/isi/
E-mail: isi@cs.vu.nl

1700 members. Organization of the world's leading statisticians.

International Thomson Publishing

(800) 354-9706
Fax (800) 487-8488
http://www.thomson.com/

Statistical books, such as Kleinbaum's *Applied Regression Analysis and Other Multivariable Methods*.

Internet Grateful Med

See National Library of Medicine.

Internet Providers: the Master List

http://www.thelist.com/

List of Internet service providers.

Internet Public Library: Reference Center

http://ipl.sils.umich.edu/ref/Center.html

Online references.

Internet Searching

°http://www.clark.net/pub/lschank/web/search.html

Advice on using the Internet.

Iowa State University Press

(800) 862-6657
(515) 292-0155
(515) 292-0140
http://aaup.pupress.princeton.edu

Association of the American University Press. Books, such as Snedecor's classic *Statistical Methods*.

JAMA (Journal of the American Medical Association)

(312) 464-5000
Sub (800) 262-2350
°http://www.ama-assn.org/

Searchable database.

John Wiley & Sons, Inc.

(800) 225-5945
http://www.wiley.com/

Online catalog of statistics books, such as Fleiss's *Statistical Methods for Rates and Proportions* and Hosmer's *Applied Logistic Regression*.

Johns Hopkins University, Baltimore

(410) 516-8000
(410) 955-3182
Medical School (410) 955-5000
(410) 955-4452
Bayview Medical Center (410) 555-0100
Department of Biostatistics (410) 955-3067
Graduate summer program in epidemiology (410) 955-7158
http://www.welch.jhu.edu/

http://www.jhbmc.jhu.edu/
°http://infonet.welch.jhu.edu/
°http://www.medbooks.jhu.edu/
http://www.sph.jhu.edu/biostats/
http://www.sph.jpu.edu/departments/epi/summer.
html

> Hospital ranked #1 in 1997 by USN&WR.
> Medical and statistical books available from
> the Medical Book Center.

Johnson & Johnson

(908) 874-1000
http://www.jnj.com/home.html

> One of the world's largest and most compre-
> hensive manufacturer of health care products.

Joint Commission on Accreditation of Health-care Organizations (JCAHO)

(708) 916-5600
(708) 916-5632
http://www.jcaho.org

Jones and Bartlett

(800) 832-0034
http://www.infoatjbpub.com

> Books, including St. James and Spiro's *Writ-
> ing and Speaking for Excellence: A Guide for
> Physicians.*

Journal of the American College of Cardiology (JACC)

(415) 759-4185
http://www.acc.org (click on JACC)

Journal of Bone and Joint Surgery

(617) 449-9780
+44-171-782-0010
http://www.jbjs.org/ (American edition)
http://www.jbjs.co.uk (British edition)

Journal of Clinical Investigation

(313) 647-8140
http://www.jci.org/

Journal of Clinical Psychiatry

(901) 751-3800
http://www.psychiatrist.com

Journal of Family Practice

(203) 406-4500

http://www.phymac.med.wayne.edu/jfp/JFP.htm

> Online resources for family physicians.

Journal of Investigative Medicine

(609) 848-1000
http://www.slackinc.com/general/jim/jimhome.htm

Journal of Medical Microbiology

+44 (0)171 976 1260
http://www.chaphall.com/chaphall/journals.html

Journal of Medical Practice

(800) 638-6423
http://www.wwilkins.com

Journal of Orthopaedic Trauma

(813) 253-2068
http://www.lrpub.com/journals/j1031.htm
E-mail: joteditor@aol.com

Journal of Respiratory Diseases

(203) 661-0600

Journal of Rheumatology

(416) 967-5155
http://www.jrheum.com

Journal of Statistical Software

(310) 825-9550
http://www.stat.ucla.edu/journals/jss/

Journal Watch

(617) 843-6356
(800) 843-6356
http://www.jwatch.org/
E-mail: jwatch@world.std.com

> Newsletter and audio tapes summarize jour-
> nal articles.

Kellogg (W.K.) Foundation

(616) 968-1611
http://www.wkkf.org/

> Grant information.

Klemtner Healthcare

See Resource Group.

Knight-Ridder Information, Inc.

(800) 334-2564

(415) 254-8800
http://www.krinfo.com
°http://www.dialog.com/

> Resources for medical researchers, *New York Times* searches, and science databases. They acquired BRS and changed their name from Dialog.

Lancet

UK +44 (0)171-436-4981
Fax +44 (0)171-436-7550
US (212) 633-3800
Fax (212) 633-3850
http://www.thelancet.com
E-mail: lanceteditorial@elsevier.co.uk

> International journal of medical science and practice.

Lenox Hill Hospital

(212) 434-2000
http://www.doctorline.com/lenox.htm

> Major teaching affiliate of New York University Medical Center.

LEXIS-NEXIS

(800) 543-6862
Sales (800) 528-1891
Express (800) 843-6476
(513) 865-6800 ext. 5505
°http://www.lexis-nexis.com/

> Information and document delivery service. Many full-text medical journals.

Lilly Endowment Inc.

(317) 924-5471

> Grant information.

Lippincott-Raven Publishers

(800) 777-2295
(301) 714-2343
http://www.lrpub.com/

> Medical and nursing books and journals, including Polit-O'Hara's *Nursing Research: Principles and Methods* and the journal *Internet Medicine*.

List of Electronic Publications

http://www.cc.emory.edu/WHSCL/medweb.ejs.html

> Part of MedWeb. Includes journal clubs.

List of Journals Indexed in Index Medicus

See National Library of Medicine.

Little, Brown and Company

(800) 343-9204
(800) 638-3030
(800) 289-6299
(617) 859-5549
(301) 714-2343 (Outside U.S.)
http://www.littlebrown.com
E-mail: lbrown@shore.net

> Books, such as Sackett's *Clinical Epidemiology: A Basic Science for Clinical Medicine* and Rothman's *Modern Epidemiology*.

Lotus/Desktop Products

See IBM.

MacArthur (John D. and Catherine T.) Foundation

(312) 726-8000
http://www.macfdn.org/

> Grant information.

Macmillan Publishing Company

(800) 223-2336
http://www.mcp.com/
http://www.mcp.com/cgi-bin/do-bookstore.cgi

> Comprehensive catalog of books.

Massachusetts General Hospital

(617) 762-2000
http://www.mgh.harvard.edu

> Hospital ranked #3 in 1997 by USN&WR.

Massachusetts Institute of Technology (MIT)

(617) 253-1000
http://web.mit.edu/

Massachusetts Medical Society

(800) 843-6356
Fax (617) 893-7368
http://www.massmed.org

> *New England Journal of Medicine* and other information services.

Material Safety Data Sheets Searches

http://research.nwfsc.noaa.gov/msds.html

Part of the US Department of Commerce. Searches for information by chemical names.

Mathematical Association of America

(202) 387-5200
(800) 331-1622
(301) 617-7800
Fax (301) 206-9789
http://www.maa.org/
E-mail: maahq@maa.org

32,000 members. Information on membership, job information, and publications.

MathSoft

(800) 569-0123
(206) 283-8802
(301) 617-7800
Fax (301) 206-9789
http://www.mathsoft.com/splus.html

S-PLUS data analysis software, customized routines, and a survival analysis tool kit.

Mayfield Publishing Company

(800) 433-1279
(415) 960-3222

Textbooks, such as Kuzma's *Basic Statistics for the Health Sciences.*

Mayo Clinic

(507) 284-2511
(507) 633-4567
(507) 284-2094
°http://www.mayo.edu/
http://www.mayo.edu/toc.html

Hospital ranked #2 in 1997 by USN&WR. Interesting information and publications for researchers. MDs, DOs, and third- and fourth-year medical students in the US may qualify for a free subscription to the journal *Mayo Clinic Proceedings.* (201) 782-5714

McAfee

+353 1 2940440
http://www.systemhouse.com/

Viruscan antivirus software.

McGraw-Hill Companies

(800) 262-4729
(212) 512-6552
(212) 512-2000
(800) 221-2956
http://www.mcgraw-hill.com

Books, such as Friedman's *Primer of Epidemiology.*

M.D. Computing

(800) 777-4643 ext. 575
(800) SPRINGER
http://enterprise.bih.harvard.edu/md-computing/

MedAccess

(617) 863-8588
http://www.medaccess.com

Physician locator, journal articles, questions and answers, and online discussions.

Med Help International

(407) 253-9048
http://medhlp.netusa.net/index.html
E-mail: staff@medhelp.netusa.net

Nonprofit medical information broker.

Medical Illustrators' Home Page

(813) 521-1143
Fax (813) 522-5022
http://medartist.com
E-mail: segilbert@earthlink.net

Resource for finding a freelance medical artist.

Medical Information Bureau

(617) 426-3660

Medical reports from 750 insurance companies. Medical reports available for approximately $8.

Medical Library Association

(312) 419-8950
http://www.kumc.edu/MLA/

Programs, conferences, and membership information.

Medical Matrix

(800) 257-8290
°http://www.medmatrix.org

Evaluation of health science resources on the Internet, including the *Hancock List and Guide to Internet Clinical Medicine Resources.*

Medical Reporter

(303) 337-6299
Fax (303) 337-9201

http://www.dash.com/netro/nwx/tmr/tmr.html
E-mail: jcooper@medreport.com

Free monthly educational health online magazine for health care consumers.

Medicine OnLine

(203) 375-7300
Fax (203) 375-6699
http://www.meds.com
E-mail: comcowic@meds.com

Cancer-related educational material.

MEDIS

See LEXIS-NEXIS.

MEDLARS

See National Library of Medicine.

Med Nexus

http://www.mednexus.com/
E-mail: ajs@mednexus.com

Medical news.

MedScape, Inc.

(212) 714-1740
°http://www.medscape.com/
E-mail: stephen_smith@medscape.com

Resources for health professionals. MEDLINE searching, textbooks, and quizzes.

MedSeek Physician Database

http://medseek.com
E-mail: info@medseek.com

Internet directory of several hundred thousand physicians.

Medtronic

(612) 574-4000
(800) 328-0810
(612) 572-5000
http://www.medtronic.com/

Medical technology company.

MedWeb: Biomedical Internet Resources

°http://www.cc.emory.edu/WHSCL/medweb.html

Provided by Emory University Health Sciences Center Library. List of links for medical researchers.

Mellon (Andrew W.) Foundation

(212) 838-8400
http://www.mellon.org/

Grant information.

Memorial Sloan-Kettering Cancer Center

(212) 639-2000
°http://www.mskcc.org

Hospital ranked #10 in 1996 by USN&WR. Cancer care and research information.

Merck & Company

(800) 659-6598
(732) 594-4000
(732) 388-9778
(732) 594-4600 (Publishing)
°http://www.merck.com

Information on drugs, jobs, and products. Access to the *Merck Manual*.

Merriam-Webster, Inc.

(800) 828-1880
http://www-lj.eb.com

Online bookstore. *Encyclopedia Britannica* online.

MetaCrawler

http://www.metacrawler.com/

Tool for searching the Internet.

Microcal Software, Inc.

(800) 969-7720
http://www.microcal.com

Original technical graphics and data analysis software.

Microsoft

Microsoft network (800) 386-5550
Tech support (206) 635-7056
°http://www.microsoft.com
http://library.microsoft.com/
°http://www.slate.com/

Software news, Microsoft library, and *Slate* magazine.

MINITAB, Inc.

(814) 238-3280
(800) 448-3555
http://www.minitab.com/

All-in-one statistical software package especially good for quality control.

Misco

(800) 876-4726

Mail-order office supplies.

MIT Press

(617) 625-8569
http://www-mitpress.mit.edu/bookstore.html

Bookstore for science, computer, and technology topics.

Morbidity and Mortality Weekly Report (MMWR)

(800) 843-6356
Sub (202) 512-1800
Editor (404) 332-4555
°http://www.cdc.gov/epo/mmwr/mmwr.html
E-mail: lists@list.cdc.gov

Electronic version of the MMWR published by the Centers for Disease Control and Prevention. Send the E-mail message "subscribe mmwr-toc" and the MMWR will be E-mailed to you each Friday.

Mosby-Year Book, Inc.

(800) 426-4545
(314) 872-8370
http://www.mosby.com/

Catalog of medical and nursing books.

Motorola Computer Systems

(800) 759-1107 ext. TLC
http://www.mot.com/

Electronic, computer, and communication equipment.

Multimedia Medical Reference Library (MMRL)

°http://www.med-library.com

Medical information, images, and sounds for physicians and patients. MEDLINE access.

National Academy of Sciences (NAS)

(202) 334-2000
http://www.nas.edu
E-mail: nasmembr@nas.edu

Honorary society with 1743 members. Listing of jobs and books. Also the home page

for the National Academy of Engineering, the Institute of Medicine, and the National Research Council.

National Association of Science Writers, Inc. (NASW)

(516) 757-5664
Fax (516) 757-0069
http://www.nasw.org

Information on books, seminars, and conferences.

National Cancer Institute

(301) 496-5583
(301) 496-9096
http://www.nci.nih.gov/

Part of the US Public Health Service/ National Institutes of Health (US PHS NIH)

National Center for Biotechnology Information (NCBI)

(301) 496-2475
http://www.ncbi.nlm.nih.gov/

Data from the National Institutes of Health/National Library of Medicine on molecular biology. Entrez, GenBank (National Institutes of Health DNA sequence database), and other resources and news.

National Center for Health Statistics

(301) 436-8500
http://www.cdc.gov/nchswww/nchshome.htm

Department of the Centers for Disease Control and Prevention.

National Center for Health Statistics' National Death Index (NDI)

(301) 436-8951
http://www.cdc.gov/nchswww/about/otheract/ndi/ndi.htm

Database to help researchers with patient follow-up information. For information on cost, a user's manual, and an application, write to: National Death Index, Division of Vital Statistics, National Center for Health Statistics, 6525 Belcrest Road, Room 840, Hyattsville, MD 20782.

National Health Care Skill Standards Project

Fax (415) 241-2702
http://www.fwl.org/nhcssp/health.html

Information on skills standards for health care workers developed by a collaboration of organizations.

National Health Information Center (NHIC)

(800) 336-4797
(301) 565-4167
http://nhic-nt.health.org/

Health information referral service.

National Information Center on Health Services (Research and Health Care Technology)

(301) 496-0176
(800) 272-4787 then: 1, 6, 3, 2
°http://www.nlm.nih.gov/nichsr/nichsr.html

National Library of Medicine program to improve the use of health information.

National Institute of Environmental Health Sciences

http://www.niehs.nih.gov/
E-mail: Rozier@niehs.nih.gov

Research on the relationship between the environment and human disease.

National Institute of General Medical Sciences

(301) 496-7301
http://www.nih.gov:80/nigms/

Agency of the National Institutes of Health. Promotes basic biomedical research that is not related to a specific disease.

National Institute for Occupational Safety and Health (NIOSH)

(800) 356-4674
http://www.cdc.gov/niosh/homepage.html
http://www.cdc.gov/diseases/niosh.html

Brochures, videos, CD-ROMs, and fact sheets.

National Institutes of Health (NIH)

(301) 496-4000
°http://www.nih.gov/
http://helix.nih.gov:8001/oe/

Main medical research organization of the US government. Resources for medical researchers. Supports more than 25,000 research projects. News, grants, resources, links to other sites, and information on research and training opportunities.

National Library of Medicine (NLM)

(800) 272-4787
(301) 496-6095
(301) 496-6193
To order Grateful Med (800) 423-9255
Assistance with searches (800) 638-8480
http://www.nlm.nih.gov/
http://www.ncbi.nlm.nih.gov/PubMed/
°http://igm.nlm.nih.gov
°http://text.nlm.nih.gov/ftrs/gateway
°http://www.nlm.nih.gov/tsd/serials/lji.html
°http://igm.nlm.nih.gov/

MEDLARS computerized system of databases, PubMed, and Grateful Med software for literature searching of MEDLINE. Other databases, such as Health Hotlines, NLM DIRLINE Database, and Toxnet. Health Services/Technology Assessment Text (HSTAT) is part of the National Library of Medicine that links to National Institutes of Health resources. *List of Journals Indexed in Index Medicus.* Internet Grateful Med.

National Network of Libraries of Medicine

(800) 338-7657
http://www.nnlm.nlm.nih.gov/

Part of the National Library of Medicine. Convenient access to health information.

National Organization for Rare Disorders, Inc. (NORD)

(800) 999-6673
(203) 746-6518
http://www.nord-rdb.com/~orphan/

Nonprofit organization that provides reports on more than 1100 rare disorders. Networking system, support groups, and a book and journal on rare disorders.

National Research Council

(202) 334-2000
http://www.nas.edu

9500 members. Advisor to the US federal government.

National Science Foundation

(703) 306-1182
(703) 306-1234
http://www.nsf.gov/

> Independent agency of the US government. Databases, survey results, studies, and grant information.

Nature

Sub (800) 524-0384
+44(0) 171 843 4985
+44(0) 171 833 4000
°http://www.america.nature.com/
http://www.nature.com/
E-mail: nature@nature.com

> International weekly science journal. Science news, events, and job information.

Nature Genetics

(202) 626-2513
(202) 626-0870
Fax (202) 626-0970
http://genetics.nature.com
E-mail: natgen@naturedc.com

> Journal.

NCBI

See National Center for Biotechnology Information.

Netlib

http://www.netlib.org/

> Mathematical software, papers, and databases.

Netscape Communications

(415) 997-3777
http://home.netscape.com

> Information on the Internet and their software, Netscape Navigator.

Network, Inc.

(518) 783-8630

> Health economics consulting firm.

Neurosciences on the Internet

http://www.neuroguide.com

New England Computer Group

(203) 431-9300
http://www.necgnet.com

> Computer consulting firm.

New England Epidemiology Institute

(617) 244-1200
Fax (617) 244-9669
http://epidemiology.com/
E-mail: epidemiol@aol.com

> Summer educational programs.

New England Journal of Medicine

(617) 893-3800
Books (800) 843-6356
Fax (617) 893-0413
°http://www.nejm.org/

> Famous journal and information on upcoming medical meetings and jobs.

New York Academy of Sciences (NYAS)

(800) 843-6927
(212) 838-0230
Fax (212) 888-2894
http://www.nyas.org

> 46,000 members. *Annals of the New York Academy of Sciences.* Promotes science and technology.

New York Medical College

(914) 594-4000
Department of Community and Preventive Medicine (914) 594-4253
Department of Health Quantitative Sciences (914) 594-4817
http://www.nymc.edu/

New York State Department of Health

(518) 473-1809
http://www.health.state.ny.us/

> Health statistics for New York.

New York Times

(212) 556-1234
http://www.nytimes.com
http://www.yourhealthdaily.com
http://www.computernewsdaily.com
http://nytsyndicate.com

See Knight-Ridder Information, Inc., for information on searching past issues.

New York University Medical Center

(212) 263-7300
°http://www.med.nyu.edu/

Grant information, educational resources, seminars, conferences, and patient information.

Niles & Associates, Inc.

(510) 559-8592
(800) 554-3049
http://www.niles.com

Software for importing, formatting, and organizing bibliographic references, such as EndNote and EndLink.

NLM

See National Library of Medicine.

Nobel Foundation

+46-8-6630920
Fax +46-8-6603847
http://www.nobel.se/

Information on the Nobel Prize and Laureates.

Nobel Prize Internet Archive

http://www.almaz.com/nobel/
http://mgm.mit.edu:8080/pevzner/Nobel.html

Interesting information, but not affiliated with the Nobel Foundation.

NTC Business Books

(800) 323-4900

See American Marketing Association.

Nursing98 (title changes each year)

(215) 646-8700
(800) 346-7844
http://www.springnet.com

Largest nursing journal, with 444,000 paid subscribers. Reference library, nursing books, sample journals, and continuing education.

Nursing Times

(071) 370-0970
Fax (071) 497-2664

Journal.

Obstetrics and Gynecology

(212) 989-5800
Fax (310) 208-2838
http://www.elsevier.com

Journal.

Occupational Safety and Health Administration (OSHA)

(202) 523-8151
http://www.osha.gov/

Part of the US Department of Labor. Statistics on safety for various occupations.

Office of Technology Assessment

http://www.wws.princeton.edu/~ota/

Provided science and technology recommendations to the US Congress for 23 years. Closed as of September 29, 1995.

Online Computer Library Center, Inc. (OCLC)

(800) 848-5800
(614) 764-6000
http://www.oclc.org/

Electronic journals online.

Oryx Press

(800) 279-6799
(602) 265-2651
Fax (800) 279-4663
Fax (602) 265-6250
°http://www.oryxpress.com
E-mail: info@oryxpress.com

Books such as Day's *How to Write and Publish a Scientific Paper.*

Ovid Technologies, Inc.

(800) 289-4277
(212) 563-3006
Fax (212) 563-3784
°http://www.ovid.com/
E-mail: sales@ovid.com

Literature searching and full-text databases that include *JAMA* and JWAT (Journal Watch).

Oxford University Press, Inc. (USA)

(800)451-7556
(212) 726-6000
(212) 726-6063
°http://www.oup-USA.org/

Publisher of more than 3000 books per year, such as Last's *A Dictionary of Epidemiology*.

Packard (David and Lucile) Foundation

(415) 948-7658
http://www.packfound.org
http://www.packard.org/

Grant information.

PaperChase

(800) 722-2075
(617) 667-5610
°http://www.paperchase.com

MEDLINE literature searching service from Beth Israel Hospital.

Papyrus Bibliography System

See Research Software Design.

PC Magazine

(800) 289-0429
°http://www.pcmag.com

Leading computer journal. Hardware and software reviews.

PDR

See Physicians' Desk Reference.

Pepi

See Epi Info, USD, Inc.

Pergamon Press

See Elsevier Publishing Company.

Personal Bibliographic Software, Inc.

See Research Information Systems.

Pew Charitable Trusts

(215) 575-9050
http://www.pewtrusts.com/

Grant information.

Pfizer

(800) 438-1985
http://www.pfizer.com

Pharmaceutical company.

Pharmaceutical Information Network

(512) 320-1600
(916) 557-1177
http://www.pharminfo.com/pin_hp.html

Comprehensive databases of drug information. FAQ. Comprehensive directory of links, forums, databases, and resources.

PhoneDisc

(800) 284-8353
http://www.dda-inc.com

CD-ROM phone book of the US.

Physicians Choice

http://www.mdchoice.com/

Evaluation of Internet sites.

Physicians' Desk Reference (PDR)

(800) 737-9206
(800) 232-7379
(800) MED-SHOP
(201) 357-7200
Fax (515) 284-6714
http://www.medec.com/
http://www.pdrbookstore.com

Physicians' GenRx

(212) 751-8033
(800) 626-3516
http://www.genrx.com/mosby/phygenrx/

Mosby's complete drug reference.

Physicians' Network

http://www.njnet.com/~embbs/pn.html

Information for physicians and health care professionals, including job listings, E-mail addresses, x-rays, and resident's forum.

Physicians' Online (POL)

(800) 332-0009
°http://www.po.com/

> MEDLINE access, drug interaction information, and medical news.

PKWARE, Inc.

(414) 354-8699
Fax (414) 354-8559
http://www.pkware.com
http://www.winzip.com

> Information on the latest version of PKZIP and Win Zip compression software, which are useful, but can be hard to find.

Planetree Health Resource Center

(415) 923-3680
Fax (415) 673-2629
http://www.ihr.com/planetre.html
E-mail: dakini@class.org

> Online medical information broker. Literature searches for a fee ($35–$100).

Poison Control Centers

(800) 343-2722
http://www.nlu.edu/aapcc
AAPCC on the Web

> List of US poison control centers. Also see the back of the PDR.

Postgraduate Medicine

(609) 426-5523
(612) 835-3222
Editor (612) 835-3222
http://www.postgradmed.com

> Journal for primary care physicians. Pearls are worth reading.

Power Point

See Microsoft

Prentice Hall Direct

(800) 922-0579
(800) 223-1360
http://w3.phdirect.com/phdirect/
Online catalog of health books.

Princeton University

(609) 258-3008
Department of Mathematics (609) 258-3034

http://www.princeton.edu
http://www.math.princeton.edu/

ProCite and Biblio-Link Package

See Research Information Systems.

Prodigy Internet

(800) 776-3449
(800) 822-6922
http://www.prodigy.com

> Online services.

Random House

(800) 726-0600
(800) 793-2665
(410) 848-1900
http://www.randomhouse.com

> Books such as the *Random House College Thesaurus.*

Raven Press

See Lippincott-Raven Publishers.

Reed Reference Publishing

(800) 521-8110
UMI (800) 521-0600
(800) 323-3288
http://www.reedref.com

> *Ulrich's International Periodicals Directory* and information on journals, such as circulation size.

Reference Manager

See Institute for Scientific Information, Inc. or Research Information Systems.

RefSys and AutoBiblio

See Biosoft.

Research! America

(800) 366-2873
(703) 739-2577
Fax (703) 739-2372
http://www.nicom.com/~ramerica/

> Organization whose mission is to make medical research a higher national priority.

Research Funding Opportunities and Administration

http://tram.rice.edu/TRAM/
E-mail: sdc@rice.edu

Searchable database of research funding sources.

Research Information Systems

(619) 438-5526
(800) 722-1227
http://www.risinc.com
http://www.procite.com/

Bibliographic reference management software for scientists, researchers, and librarians, including Reference Manager, ProCite, and Biblio-Link.

Research Software Design

(503) 796-1368
http://www.rsd.com/~rsd/
E-mail: sales@rsd.com

Papyrus Personal Bibliographic Database System software to computerize references.

Resource Group

(212) 463-5024
Fax (212) 463-3456
http://www.klemtner.com

Health care education and communication, pharmaceutical advertising, and marketing expertise.

Reuters Health Information Services

(212) 603-3300
*http://www.reutershealth.com/

Latest health news and classified advertisements.

Rhône-Poulenc Rorer

(610) 454-8000
http://www.rpr.rpna.com/

RN (Registered Nurse)

(201) 358-7477
(201) 358-7200

Journal.

Robert Wood Johnson Foundation

(609) 452-8701
http://www.rwjf.org/maim.html

Largest US philanthropy devoted to health and health care.

Running Press

(800) 345-5359

Books, such as *Gray's Anatomy*.

Salk Institute for Biological Studies

(619) 453-4100
http://www.salk.edu

News about research and job opportunities.

Sample Size Software

(604) 822-0975
*http://www.interchg.ubc.ca/cacb/power

Comprehensive list of power analysis software for microcomputers. Links to sites that provide online sample size and power calculations. Information about purchasing power analysis software.

SAS Institute Inc.

(919) 677-8000
(800) 544-6678
http://www.sas.com/

Statistical software and services.

W.B. Saunders Company

(800) 545-2522
(800) 544-6678
(215) 238-7800
http://www.wbsaunders.com/
http://customerservice.wbsaunders.com/
http://customerservice.hbpp.com/

Books, such as *Mausner's Epidemiology: An Introductory Text.*

Schering-Plough

(908) 298-4000
http://www.sch-plough.com/

Pharmaceutical company.

Science

(202) 326-6526
(202) 326-6501
*http://www.sciencemag.org/
http://www.aaas.org

Prestigious journal published by the American Association for the Advancement of Science.

Science Citation Index

See Institute for Scientific Information, Inc.

Scientist

(800) 258-6008
°http://www.the-scientist.library.upenn.edu/
http://165.123.33.33

Newspaper for life sciences professionals.

SilverPlatter Information, Inc.

(617) 769-2599
(800) 343-0064
°http://www.silverplatter.com/
http://www.silverplatter.com/physicians

MEDLINE literature searching via CD-ROM or the Internet (WebSPIRS).

Six Senses

http://www.echo-strategies.com/sixsenses/

Evaluation of Web sites.

SmithKline Beecham

(573) 635-8326
(800) 366-8900
http://www.sb.com

Information on products, services, and jobs.

Society for Clinical Trials

(410) 433-4722
Fax (410) 435-8631
http://home.aol.com/sctbalt
http://www.members.aol.com/sctbalt/index.htm
E-mail: sctbalt@aol.com

Association of experts on clinical trials.

Society for Epidemiologic Research (SER)

(410) 223-1620
(801) 581-7234
http://www.sph.jhu.edu/Info/Publications/JEPI/ser.htm

Sponsor of the *American Journal of Epidemiology* and Epidemiologic Reviews.

Society for Risk Analysis (SRA)

(703) 790-3926
(703) 790-1745
http://mijuno.larc.nasa.gov/dfc/societies/sra.html
E-mail: sraburkmgt@aol.com

Risk Analysis Journal.

Society for Scholarly Publishing

(303) 422-3914
http://www.edoc.com/ssp

Scholarly communication organization. Newsletter *Scholarly Publishing Today.*

Society for Technical Communication

(703) 522-4114
http://www.stc-va.org

20,000 technical writers, editors, and freelance consultants.

Software Publishing Corporation

(800) 336-8360
(970) 522-9064
http://www.spco.com

Harvard Graphics and other software products.

Spectratone Color Labs

(914) 946-3336
(800) 427-3336
To modem slides (914) 946-5550
Fax (914) 946-4772
http://www.spectratone.com

Traditional photographic prints and digital services, including 35-mm slides and large-format digital posters from 4 feet wide and any length.

S-PLUS

See MathSoft.

Springer Publishing Company, Inc.

(212) 431-4370
http://www.libertyweb.com/springer.html

Nursing and psychology books, such as Sheridan's *How to Write and Publish Articles in Nursing* and Barnum's *Writing and Getting Published: A Primer for Nurses.*

Springer-Verlag, New York, Inc.

(800) 777-4643
(212) 460-1682
(800) SPRINGER
http://www.springer-ny.com

Nursing and statistical books, such as Kleinbaum's *Logistic Regression: A Self-Learning Text* and Briscoe's *Preparing Scientific Illus-*

trations: A Guide to Better Posters, Presentations, and Publications.

SPSS (Statistical Products for Service Solutions—formerly Statistical Package for Social Sciences)

(800) 543-2185
(312) 329-2400
(800) 525-4974
(213) 479-7799
(310) 207-8800
SPSS Bookstore (800) 253-2565
Manuals on SPSS (800) 374-1200
Eureka! catalog (800) 621-1393
BMDP technical support (312) 467-5232
SPSS technical support (312) 329-3410
Systat technical support (312) 494-3283
°http://www.spss.com/
°http://www.spss.com/Pubs/
E-mail: support@spss.com technical support
E-mail: sales@spss.com.sales

Statistical software. Formerly Statistical Package for the Social Science. SPSS acquired several other companies that produced the statistical software packages BMDP and Systat.

St. Anthony's Publishing, Inc.

(800) 632-0123

ICD coding books.

Stanford University Hospital

(415) 723-4000
Medical School (415) 725-3900
Department of Statistics (415) 723-2625
Hospital ranked #8 in 1997 by USN&WR.
http://www-med.stanford.edu/shs/
http://med-www.stanford.edu/
http://playfair.stanford.edu

Graduate school ranked #2 in mathematical statistics in 1996 by USN&WR.

Stata Corporation

(800) 782-8272
(409) 696-4600
Fax (409) 696-4601
http://www.stata.com
E-mail: stata@stata.com

Statistical software.

State University of New York at Albany

(518) 442-3300
(518) 473-1809

Department of Mathematics and Statistics (518) 442-4602
http://www.albany.edu/
http://www.albany.edu/sph/

STATGRAPHICS

See Statistical Graphics Corporation

Statistical Assessment Service

(202) 223-3193
Fax (202) 872-4014
°http://www.stats.org
E-mail: stats2100@aol.com

Nonpartisan, nonprofit research organization to help journalists with statistical and quantitative analysis for public policy. Newsletter *STATS 2100.*

Statistical Graphics Corporation

(800) 232-7828
(609) 924-9374
http://www.sgcop.com

STATGRAPHICS software.

Statistics and Epidemiologic Research Corporation

(206) 632-3014

Statistical consulting firm for clinical trials.

StatLib

See Carnegie Mellon University.

StatSoft

(918) 749-1119
http://www.statsoftinc.com

STATISTICA data analysis software.

Stat-USA

(202) 482-2164
(800) STAT-USA
http://www.stat-usa.gov/

Business, economic, and government information for a fee from the US Department of Commerce.

Statview

(510) 540-1949
Fax (510) 540-0260
http://www.abacus.com

Statistical program.

StatXact

See Cytel Software Corporation.

Stedman's Electronic Medical Dictionary

See Williams & Wilkins.

Surgeon General

(301) 443-6496
http://www.os.dhhs.gov/progorg/ophs/

Office of the US government's top physician.

Swets & Zeitlinger

31-252-435111
(610) 644-4944
http://www.swets.nl

SWETS medical journal document delivery service and other library and publishing services.

Switchboard

http://www2.switchboard.com/

Telephone numbers and addresses of people and businesses in the US.

Systat, Inc.

See SPSS.

THOMAS

http://thomas.loc.gov/

Home page of the US Library of Congress. Information about the US Congress and American laws.

Tools & Techniques, Inc.

(800) 459-1308
http://moontowner.com/dj

Data Junction software.

Top Charitable Organizations in the US

http://206.210.73.13/library/top40.html
http://fdncenter.org/2trends/2fdgiv.html

Links to organizations that provide research grants.

Toxnet

See National Library of Medicine.

Tripod

(212) 486-3561
http://www.tripod.com

Health information for college students.

True Epistat

(800) 326-1488
(972) 680-1376
Fax (972) 680-1303

Easy-to-use statistical software for 95% confidence intervals, odds ratios, Fisher's exact test, and sample size calculations. Graphic capabilities, survival analysis, and meta-analysis.

Ulrich's International Periodicals Directory

See Reed Reference Publishing.

UMI

See University Microfilm International.

UnCover Company–Carl Corporation

(800) 787-7979
(303) 758-3030
+44-1865-261362
Fax (303) 758-5946
°http://www.carl.org/carl.html
http://www.carl.org/uncover/unchome.html
E-mail: uncover@carl.org

Popular document delivery service. Search for free; pay for article delivery. Spun off from the Colorado Alliance of Research Librarians. Now a Knight-Ridder Information Company.

UNESCO

http://www.unesco.org

United Nations Educational, Scientific and Cultural Organization.

Uniform Requirements for Manuscripts Submitted to Biomedical Journals

See International Committee of Medical Journal Editors.

United HealthCare Corporation

(612) 936-1300
http://www.uhc.com/

Subsidiary of Applied HealthCare Informatics. Software and analysis for cost-effectiveness of medical treatments.

University of California-Berkeley

(510) 643-6132
Department of Statistics (510) 642-2781
Fax (510) 642-7892
°http://stat-ftp.berkeley.edu/
Department of Statistics.

> Graduate school ranked #1 in mathematical statistics in 1996 by USN&WR. Statistical resources.

University of California-Los Angeles Medical Center

(310) 825-9111
Department of Biostatistics (310) 825-5250
http://www.mednet.ucla.edu/som/
°http://sun.sunlab.ph.ucla.edu/biostat/
http://www.stat.ucla.edu/

> Hospital ranked #5 in 1997 by USN&WR. Useful links.

°http://www.medctr.ucla.edu/

University of California-San Francisco Medical Center

(415) 476-1000
Department of Epidemiology and Biostatistics (415) 476-8671
Fax (415) 476-0868
°http://www.ucsf.edu/
°http://www.biostat.ucsf.edu

> Hospital ranked #7 in 1997 by USN&WR.

http://www.ucsf.edu/health/hospital.html/

University of Chicago Hospitals

(312) 702-8333
°http://galton.uchicago.edu

> Graduate school ranked #5 in mathematical statistics in 1996 by USN&WR. Comprehensive source of statistical information. Hospital ranked #3 in 1997 by USN&WR.

http://www.uch.uchicago.edu/

University of Chicago Press

(312) 702-7700
http://www.press.uchicago.edu

Books, such as Williams' *Style: Toward Clarity and Grace* and the *Chicago Manual of Style.*

University of Connecticut

Department of Statistics (860) 486-2008
Statistical resources (860) 486-2951
http://ruddles.stat.uconn.edu

University of Iowa Hospitals and Clinics

(319) 356-1616

> http://www.uihc.uiowa.edu/
> Hospital ranked #15 in 1997 by USN&WR.

University of Michigan Medical Center at Ann Arbor

(313) 936-4000
Fax (313) 936-9437
Center for Statistical Consultation and Research (313) 764-7828
Fax (313) 747-2240
Statistical Resources (313) 764-5451
Department of Biostatistics (313) 764-5450
Department of Statistics (313) 763-3520
http://www.med.umich.edu
http://www.umich.edu/~cscar/
http://www.sph.umich.edu/group/biostat/

> Hospital ranked #10 in 1997 by USN&WR.

University Microfilm International (UMI)

(800) 248-0360
Fax (415) 433-0100
http://www.umi.com

> InfoStore information and document delivery service, microfilm, and dissertations.

University of Pennsylvania Center for Clinical Epidemiology and Biostatistics

(215) 898-8964
http://cceb.med.upenn.edu

University of Texas-MD Anderson Cancer Center

(713) 792-6345
(713) 792-2121
Fax (713) 792-7573
http://utmdacc.mda.uth.tmc.edu
°http://utmdacc.uth.tmc.edu/

> Hospital ranked #9 in 1996 by USN&WR. Cancer resources and library.

University of Washington Medical Center, Seattle

http://www.washington.edu/medical

Hospital ranked #10 in 1997 by USN&WR.

University of Wisconsin at Madison

(608) 262-1234
(608) 262-2598
http://www.stat.wisc.edu/
http://www.biostat.wisc.edu/biostat/biostat.html

Graduate school ranked #3 in mathematical statistics in 1996 by USN&WR.

US Census Bureau

(301) 457-2135
(301) 457-2071
http://www.census.gov/

US population statistics.

US Government Printing Office

(202) 512-1800
(202) 783-3238
(202) 512-0828
Fax (202) 512-2250
http://www.access.gpo.gov/

Healthy People 2000 Report and other publications for medical researchers.

US News & World Report

(800) 836-6397
(202) 955-2000
http://www.usnews.com
http://www.usnews.com/usnews/nycu/hosphigh.htm

News magazine that ranks hospitals and graduate schools.

US Public Health Service

(301) 496-2403
(301) 690-7694
PHS Agencies (301) 690-6467
http://phs.os.dhhs.gov/phs/phs.html
http://phs.os.dhhs.gov/progorg/progorg.html
°http://phs.os.dhhs.gov/progorg/ophs/

Information on the Surgeon General and other topics.

USD

See Epi Info, USD, Inc.

Van Nostrand Reinhold

(800) 842-3636
(212) 254-3232
http://www.thomson.com/vnr.html

Books, such as Kleinbaum's *Epidemiologic Research: Principles and Quantitative Methods.*

Virtual Hospital

°http://vh.radiology.uiowa.edu

Teaching files and publications from the Department of Radiology, University of Iowa College of Medicine.

Virtual Library of Statistics

http://www.stat.ufl.edu/vlib/statistics.html

Links to statistical sites.

Virtual Medical Center

°http://www-sci.lib.uci.edu/hsg/medical.html

Links to medical teaching resources and CME courses.

Virtual Reference Desk

http://thorplus.lib.purdue.edu/reference/index.html

Resource from Purdue University. Dictionaries, telephone books, maps, zip codes, and other information.

Visible Human Project

CD-ROM version (515) 296-9908
(408) 426-2855
Dissectable human three-dimensional anatomy on CD-ROM (800) EAI-6777
http://www.nlm.nih.gov/research/visible/visible_human.html
http://www.eai.com

Online three-dimensional images of the human body.

Warner-Lambert

(201) 540-2000
http://www.warner-lambert.com/

Pharmaceutical company.

Westchester County Medical Center

(914) 285-7000
http://www.wcmc.com/

Academic referral hospital affiliated with New York Medical College.

White House

(202) 456-1111
http://www.whitehouse.gov/

Little medical information, but interesting.

WhoWhere

http://www.whowhere.com/

E-mail addresses.

Williams & Wilkins

(800) 527-5597
(410) 528-8555
(410) 528-4223
Books customer service (800) 638-0672
Electronic media (800) 527-5597
Journals customer service (800) 638-6423
Fax (410) 528-8596
°http://www.wwilkins.com
http://www.wwilkins.com/hot/stedmanelec/
index.html
E-mail: custserv@wwilkins.com

Medical books and software, including *Stedman's Medical Dictionary,* the *AMA Manual of Style,* and Hulley's *Designing Clinical Research: An Epidemiologic Approach.* Resources for medical students and a catalog to search. Stedman's Electronic Medical Dictionary and Stedman's Plus Spellchecker software.

Woodruff (Robert W.) Foundation, Inc.

(404) 522-6755

Woodward/White, Inc.

(800) 447-8438
Fax (803) 648-0300
http://www.bestdoctors.com/

Consulting firm that wrote *The Best Doctors in America.*

World Health Organization

(212) 963-4388
(919) 541-7537
+44 22/791 2111
http://www.who.ch/
gopher://gopher.who.ch

Publications, reports, medical conferences, programs, news, outbreaks, and health issues from around the world.

World Medical Association, Inc.

33 4.50 40 75 75
Fax 33 4.50 40 59 37

Declaration of Helsinki.

Writer's Digest Books

(800) 289-0963
(513) 531-2690
Fax (513) 531-4744
http://www.howdesign.com

Catalog of writing books.

WWW FAQ

http://www.boutell.com/faq/www_faq.html

Frequently asked questions about the World Wide Web. Good site for people who are learning how to access information on the Internet.

WWW Virtual Library

http://www.w3.org/vl/
http://www.ohsu.edu/cliniweb/wwwvl/

Medical information on the Internet and links to other useful sites. WWW Virtual Library: Biosciences: Medicine.

Yahoo

http://www.yahoo.com/health/medicine/

Tool to search the Internet for health-related topics. To find other search engines, use Net Search on your browser. Also try the multiple search engines, such as MetaCrawler.

Yale University

(203) 432-1333
(203) 785-2572
School of Medicine (203) 432-4771
Office of Public Information (203) 785-5824
Cushing/Whitney Medical Library
(203) 785-5824
Department of Epidemiology and Public Health
(includes Division of Biostatistics)
(203) 785-2844
Department of Statistics (203) 432-0666
http://www.yale.edu/
http://info.med.yale.edu/medical/
http://www.med.yale.edu/library/
http://www.med.yale.edu/eph/
°http://descartes.stat.yale.edu/HOME.html

World Medical Association Declaration of Helsinki

Recommendations Guiding Physicians in Biomedical Research Involving Human Subjects

INTRODUCTION

It is the mission of the physician to safeguard the health of the people. His or her knowledge and conscience are dedicated to the fulfillment of this mission.

The Declaration of Geneva of the World Medical Association binds the physician with the words, "The health of my patient will be my first consideration," and the International Code of Medical Ethics declares that, "A physician shall act only in the patient's interest when providing medical care which might have the effect of weakening the physical and mental condition of the patient."

The purpose of biomedical research involving human subjects must be to improve diagnostic, therapeutic and prophylactic procedures and the understanding of the aetiology and pathogenesis of disease.

In current medical practice most diagnostic, therapeutic or prophylactic procedures involve hazards. This applies especially to biomedical research.

Medical progress is based on research which ultimately must rest in part on experimentation involving human subjects.

In the field of biomedical research a fundamental distinction must be recognized between medical research in which the aim is essentially diagnostic or therapeutic for a patient, and medical research, the essential object of which is purely scientific and without implying direct diagnostic or therapeutic value to the person subjected to the research.

Special caution must be exercised in the conduct of research which may affect the environment, and the welfare of animals used for research must be respected.

Because it is essential that the results of laboratory experiments be applied to human beings to further scientific knowledge and to help suffering humanity, the World Medical Association has prepared the following recommendations as a guide to every physician in biomedical research involving human subjects. They should be kept under review in the future. It must be stressed that the standards as drafted are only a guide to physicians all over the world. Physicians are not relieved from criminal, civil, and ethical responsibilities under the laws of their own countries.

I. BASIC PRINCIPLES

1. Biomedical research involving human subjects must conform to generally accepted scientific principles and should be based on adequately performed labora-

Adopted by the 18th World Medical Assembly, Helsinki, Finland, 1964, and amended by the 29th World Medical Assembly, Tokyo, Japan, 1975; 35th World Medical Assembly, Venice, Italy, 1983; 41st World Medical Assembly, Hong Kong, 1989; and the 48th General Assembly, Somerset West, Republic of South Africa, 1996. Reprinted with permission from the World Medical Association.

tory and animal experimentation and on a thorough knowledge of the scientific literature.

2. The design and performance of each experimental procedure involving human subjects should be clearly formulated in an experimental protocol which should be transmitted for consideration, comment and guidance to a specially appointed committee independent of the investigator and the sponsor provided that this independent committee is in conformity with the laws and regulations of the country in which the research experiment is performed.

3. Biomedical research involving human subjects should be conducted only by scientifically qualified persons and under the supervision of a clinically competent medical person. The responsibility for the human subject must always rest with a medically qualified person and never rest on the subject of the research, even though the subject has given his or her consent.

4. Biomedical research involving human subjects cannot legitimately be carried out unless the importance of the objective is in proportion to the inherent risk to the subject.

5. Every biomedical research project involving human subjects should be preceded by careful assessment of predictable risks in comparison with foreseeable benefits to the subject or to others. Concern for the interests of the subject must always prevail over the interests of science and society.

6. The right of the research subject to safeguard his or her integrity must always be respected. Every precaution should be taken to respect the privacy of the subject and to minimize the impact of the study on the subject's physical and mental integrity and on the personality of the subject.

7. Physicians should abstain from engaging in research projects involving human subjects unless they are satisfied that the hazards involved are believed to be predictable. Physicians should cease any investigation if the hazards are found to outweigh the potential benefits.

8. In publication of the results of his or her research, the physician is obliged to preserve the accuracy of the results. Reports of experimentation not in accordance with the principles laid down in this Declaration should not be accepted for publication.

9. In any research on human beings, each potential subject must be adequately informed of the aims, methods, anticipated benefits and potential hazards of the study and the discomfort it may entail. He or she should be informed that he or she is at liberty to abstain from participation in the study and that he or she is free to withdraw his or her consent to participation at any time. The physician should then obtain the subject's freely given informed consent, preferably in writing.

10. When obtaining informed consent for the research project the physician should be particularly cautious if the subject is in a dependent relationship to him or her or may consent under duress. In that case the informed consent should be obtained by a physician who is not engaged in the investigation and who is completely independent of this official relationship.

11. In case of legal incompetence, informed consent should be obtained from the legal guardian in accordance with national legislation. Where physical or mental incapacity makes it impossible to obtain informed consent, or when the subject is a minor, permission from the responsible relative replaces that of the subject in accordance with national legislation. Whenever the minor child is in fact able to give a consent, the minor's consent must be obtained in addition to the consent of the minor's legal guardian.

12. The research protocol should always contain a statement of the ethical considerations involved and should indicate that the principles enunciated in the present Declaration are complied with.

II. MEDICAL RESEARCH COMBINED WITH PROFESSIONAL CARE (CLINICAL RESEARCH)

1. In the treatment of the sick person, the physician must be free to use a new diagnostic and therapeutic measure, if in his or her judgment it offers hope of saving life, reestablishing health or alleviating suffering.

2. The potential benefits, hazards and discomfort of a new method should be weighed against the advantages of the best current diagnostic and therapeutic methods.

3. In any medical study, every patient—including those of a control group, if any—should be assured of the best proven diagnostic and therapeutic method. This does not exclude the use of inert placebo in studies where no proven diagnostic or therapeutic method exists.

4. The refusal of the patient to participate in a study must never interfere with the physician–patient relationship.

5. If the physician considers it essential not to obtain informed consent, the specific reasons for this proposal should be stated in the experimental protocol for transmission to the independent committee (I,2).

6. The physician can combine medical research with professional care, the objective being the acquisition of new medical knowledge, only to the extent that medical research is justified by its potential diagnostic or therapeutic value for the patient.

III. NON-THERAPEUTIC BIOMEDICAL RESEARCH INVOLVING HUMAN SUBJECTS

(Non-Clinical Biomedical Research)

1. In the purely scientific application of medical research carried out on a human being, it is the duty of the physician to remain the protector of the life and health of that person on whom biomedical research is being carried out.

2. The subjects should be volunteers—either healthy persons or patients for whom the experimental design is not related to the patient's illness.

3. The investigator or the investigating team should discontinue the research if in his/her or their judgment it may, if continued, be harmful to the individual.

4. In research on man, the interest of science and society should never take precedence over considerations related to the well-being of the subject.

Ode to Multiauthorship:
A Multicentre, Prospective Random Poem

All cases complete, the study was over
the data were entered, lost once, and recovered.
Results were greeted with considerable glee
p value (two-tailed) equalling 0.0493.
The severity of illness, oh what a discovery,
was inversely proportional to the chance of recovery.
When the paper's first draft had only begun
the wannabe authors lined up one by one.
To jockey for their eternal positions
(for who would be first, second, and third)
and whom "et aled" in all further citations.
Each centre had seniors, each senior ten bees,
the bees had technicians and nurses to please.
The list it grew longer and longer each day,
as new authors appeared to enter the fray.
Each fought with such fury to stake his or her place
being just a "participant" would be a disgrace.
For the appendix is piled with hundreds of others
and seen by no one but spouses and mothers.
If to "publish or perish" is how academics are bred
then to miss the masthead is near to be dead.
As the number of authors continued to grow
they outnumbered the patients by two to one or so.
While PIs faxed memos to company headquarters
the bees and the nurses took care of the orders.
They'd signed up the patients, and followed them weekly
heard their complaints, and kept casebooks so neatly.
There were seniors from centres that enrolled two or three
who threatened "foul play" if not on the marquee.
But the juniors and helpers who worked into the night
were simply "acknowledged" or left off outright.
"Calm down" cried the seniors to the quivering drones
there's place for you all on the RPU clones.
When the paper was finished and sent for review
six authors didn't know that the study was through.
Oh the work was so hard, and the fights oh so bitter
for the glory of publishing and grabbing the glitter.
Imagine the wars when in six months or better
The Editor's response, "please make it a letter."

The order of the authors is not necessarily related to specific contributions, but to the order in which each made their acquaintance with the first author. However, all have made significant contributions to the poem. The authors acknowledge their debt to Theodore Geisel. This letter was originally submitted to The Lancet as an article.

RPU=repeating publishable unit; PI=principal investigator

°*Harold W Horowitz, Nicholas H Fiebach, Stuart M Levitz, Jo Seibel, Edwin H Smail, Edward E Telzak, Gary P Wormser, Robert B Nadelman, Marisa Montecalvo, John Nowakowski, John Raffalli*

Departments of Medicine, °New York Medical College, Valhalla, New York, 10595, USA; Yale University School of Medicine, New Haven, CT; Boston University School of Medicine, Boston, MA; Metrowest Medical Center, Framingham, MA; and Albert Einstein School of Medicine, Bronx, New York

Bibliography

Abby M, Massey MD, Galandiuk S, et al. Peer review is an effective screening process to evaluate medical manuscripts. JAMA 1994;272:105–107.

Alpha-Tocopherol, Beta Carotene Cancer Prevention Study Group. The effect of vitamin E and beta carotene on the incidence of lung cancer and other cancers in male smokers. N Engl J Med 1994;330:1029–1035.

Altman DG. Practical statistics for medical research. New York: Chapman & Hall; 1991.

Altman DG, Goodman SN. Transfer of technology from statistical journals to the biomedical literature: past trends and future predictions. JAMA 1994;272:129–132.

American Heritage dictionary of the English language. 3rd ed. Boston: Houghton Mifflin; 1996.

American Psychological Association. Publication manual of the American Psychological Association. 4th ed. Washington (DC): American Psychological Association; 1994.

American Psychologist. Summary report of journal operations 1995 (archival issue). 1996;51:876–877.

Armitage P, Berry G. Statistical methods in medical research. 3rd ed. Oxford (England): Blackwell Scientific; 1994.

Babbie ER. Survey research methods. 2nd ed. Belmont (CA): International Thomson; 1990.

Bailar JC III, Mosteller F, editors. Medical uses of statistics. 2nd ed. Boston: Massachusetts Medical Society; 1992.

Baker SS. Writing nonfiction that sells. Cincinnati: Writer's Digest Books; 1986.

Barnum BS. Writing and getting published: a primer for nurses. New York: Springer; 1995.

Bartko JJ. Rationale for reporting standard deviations rather than standard errors of the mean [editorial]. Am J Psychiatry 1985;142:1060.

Berry DA. Ethics and ECMO [comment]. Stat Sci 1989;4:306–316.

Berwick DM. Quality of health care. Part 5: payment by capitation and the quality of care. N Engl J Med 1996;335:1227–1231.

Blumenthal D. Part 1: quality of care—what is it? N Engl J Med 1996;335:891–894.

Blumenthal D. Quality of health care. Part 4: the origins of the quality-of-care debate. N Engl J Med 1996;335:1146–1149.

Blumenthal D, Epstein AM. Quality of health care. Part 6: the role of physicians in the future of quality management. N Engl J Med 1996;335:1328–1331.

Brallier JM, editor. In: Cuvier G. Medical wit and wisdom: the best medical quotations from Hippocrates to Groucho Marx. Philadelphia: Running Press; 1993.

Breslow NE, Day NE. Statistical methods in cancer research. Vol. 1. The analysis of case–control studies (IARC Scientific Publications No. 32):5–338. Lyon (France): International Agency for Research on Cancer; 1980.

Breslow NE, Day NE. Statistical methods in cancer research. Vol. 2. The design and analysis of cohort studies (IARC Scientific Publications No. 82):1–406. Lyon (France): International Agency for Research on Cancer; 1987.

Briscoe MH. Preparing scientific illustrations: a guide to better posters, presentations, and publications. 2nd ed. New York: Springer-Verlag; 1996.

Brook RH, McGlynn EA, Cleary PD. Quality of health care. Part 2: measuring quality of care. N Engl J Med 1996;335:966–970.

Bulpitt CJ. Randomised controlled clinical trials. 2nd ed. Norwell (MA): Kluwer Academic Publishers; 1996.

Chassin MR. Quality of health care. Part 3: improving the quality of care. N Engl J Med 1996;335:1060–1063.

Chicago manual of style. 14th ed. Chicago: University of Chicago Press; 1993.

Clark S. Taming the marketing jungle: marketing when your creativity is high and your budget is low. Seattle: Hara; 1994.

Colton T. The 'power' of sound statistics [editorial; comment]. JAMA 1990; 263:281.

Conover WJ. Some reasons for not using the Yates continuity correction on 2×2 contingency tables. J Am Stat Assoc 1974;69:374–376.

Cox DR. Regression models and life-tables. J R Stat Soc [B] 1972;34:187–220.

Crichton M. Medical obfuscation: structure and function [sounding board]. N Engl J Med 1975;293: 1257–1259.

Daintith J, Isaacs A, editors. Medical quotes: a thematic dictionary. Oxford: Market House Books; 1989.

Dawson-Saunders B, Trapp RG. Basic and clinical biostatistics. 2nd ed. Norwalk (CT): Appleton & Lange; 1994.

Day RA. How to write and publish a scientific paper. 4th ed. Phoenix: Oryx Press; 1994.

Dean AG, Dean JA, Burton AH, Dicker RC. Epi Info. Version 6. A word processing program, database, and statistics program for public health on IBM-compatible microcomputers. Atlanta: Centers for Disease Control and Prevention; 1994.

Ewigman BG, Crane JP, Frigoletto FD, et al. Effect of prenatal ultrasound screening on perinatal outcome. N Engl J Med 1993; 329:821–827.

Falco FJE, Hennessey WJ, Goldberg G, et al. Standardized nerve conduction studies in the lower limb of the healthy elderly. Am J Phys Med Rehabil 1994;73:168–174.

Fleiss JL. Statistical methods for rates and proportions. 2nd ed. New York: John Wiley; 1981.

Fleiss JL, Tytun A, Ury HK. A simple approximation for calculating sample sizes for comparing two independent proportions. Biometrics 1980;36:343–346.

Fletcher RH, Fletcher SW, Wagner EH. Clinical epidemiology: the essentials. 3rd ed. Baltimore: Williams & Wilkins; 1996.

Fox RJ, Crask MR, Kim J. Mail survey response rate: a meta-analysis of selected techniques for inducing response. Public Opin 1988;52:467–491.

Fried C. The practice of experimentation. In: Bearn AG, Black DAK, Hiatt HH, editors. Medical experimentation: personal integrity and social policy. New York: American Elsevier; 1974. p. 158.

Friedman GD. Primer of epidemiology. 4th ed. New York: McGraw-Hill; 1994.

Gardner MJ, Altman DG. Statistics with confidence: confidence intervals and statistical guidelines. London: British Medical Journal; 1989.

Garfield E. SCI journal citation reports: a bibliographic analysis of science journals in the ISI database [printed guide to the microfiche edition]. Philadelphia: Institute for Scientific Information; 1995.

Garland J. In: Strauss MB, editor. Familiar medical quotations. Boston: Little, Brown; 1968. p. 672.

Gilmore E. 'Call me Jim': James Thurber speaking. Columbus Dispatch 1958 Aug 3; Collected in: Fensch T, editor. Conversations with James Thurber. Jackson (MI): University of Mississippi Press; 1989. p. 50.

Hall GM, editor. How to write a paper. London: British Medical Journal; 1994.

Halsey MJ. In: Hall GM, editor. How to write a paper. London: British Medical Journal; 1994.

Hill AB. The environment and disease: association or causation? Proceedings of the Royal Society of Medicine, Section on Occupational Medicine. 1965. 58; 295 pp. 7–12.

Hosmer DW Jr, Lemeshow S. Applied logistic regression. New York: John Wiley; 1989.

Hulley SB, Cummings SR, editors. Designing clinical research: an epidemiologic approach. Baltimore: Williams & Wilkins; 1988.

Huth EJ, editor. How to write and publish papers in the medical sciences. 2nd ed. Baltimore: Williams & Wilkins; 1990.

Huth EJ, Style Manual Committee, Council of Biology Editors. Scientific style and format: the CBE manual for authors, editors and publishers. 6th ed. New York: Cambridge University Press; 1994.

Ingelfinger JA, Mosteller F, Thibodeau LA, Ware JH. Biostatistics in clinical medicine. 3rd ed. New York: McGraw-Hill; 1994.

International Committee of Medical Journal Editors. Uniform requirements for manuscripts submitted to biomedical journals. N Engl J Med 1997;336:309–315.

International Conference on Harmonisation. Guidelines on structure and content of clinical study reports. Federal Register 1996;61:37319–37343.

Iverson C, Dan BB, Glitman P, et al. The American Medical Association manual of style. 8th ed. Baltimore: Williams & Wilkins; 1989.

Kaplan EL, Meier P. Nonparametric estimation from incomplete observations. J Am Stat Assoc 1958;53:457–481.

Kassirer JP, Angell M. Redundant publication: a reminder (not to publish repetitive data) [editorial]. N Engl J Med 1995;333:449–450.

Kassirer JP, Campion EW. Peer review: crude and understudied, but indispensable. JAMA 1994;272: 96–97.

Kleinbaum DG. Applied regression analysis and other multivariable methods. 2nd ed. Belmont (CA): International Thomson; 1988.

Kleinbaum DG. Logistic regression: a self-learning text. New York: Springer-Verlag; 1995.

Kleinbaum DG, Kupper LL, Morgenstern H. Epidemiologic research: principles and quantitative methods. New York: Van Nostrand; 1982.

Kleinbaum DG, Kupper LL, Muller KE. Applied regression analysis and other multivariable methods. 2nd ed. Boston: PWS-Kent; 1988.

Kuzma JW. Basic statistics for the health sciences. 2nd ed. Mountain View (CA): Mayfield; 1992.

Last JM. A dictionary of epidemiology. 3rd ed. New York: Oxford University Press; 1995.

Lee ET. Statistical methods for survival data analysis. 2nd ed. New York: John Wiley; 1992.

Liggins GC, Howie RN. A controlled trial of antepartum glucocorticoid treatment for prevention of the respiratory distress syndrome in premature infants. Pediatrics 1972;50:515–525.

Lipsitz SR, Fitzmaurice GM, Orav EJ, et al. Performance of generalized estimating equations in practical situations. Biometrics 1994;50:270–278.

Lock SP. The future of medical journals. In: Commemoration of 150 years of the British Medical Journal. London: British Medical Journal; 1991.

Mann HB, Whitney DR. On a test of whether one of two random variables is stochastically larger than the other. Ann Math Stat 1947;18:50–60.

Mantel N, Haenszel W. Statistical aspects of the analysis of data from retrospective studies of disease. J Natl Cancer Inst 1959;22:719–748.

Marantz PR. Beta carotene, vitamin E, and lung cancer [letter; comment]. N Engl J Med 1994;331: 611–614.

Mausner JS, Kramer S. Epidemiology: an introductory text. 2nd ed. Philadelphia: WB Saunders; 1985.

Mehta CR, Patel NR, Gray R. Computing an exact confidence interval for the common odds ratio in several 2 × 2 contingency tables. J Am Stat Assoc 1985;80:969–973.

Merriam-Webster's collegiate dictionary. 10th ed. Springfield (MA): Merriam-Webster; 1993.

Morton RF, Hebel JR. A study guide to epidemiology and biostatistics. 3rd ed. Gaithersburg (MD): Aspen; 1990.

Moses LE, Emerson JD, Hosseini H. Analyzing data from ordered categories. N Engl J Med 1984;311:442–448.

Naber SP, Tsutsumi Y, Yin S, et al. Strategies for the analysis of oncogene overexpression: studies of the *neu* oncogene in breast carcinoma. Am J Clin Pathol 1990;94:125–136.

National Center for Health Statistics. User's manual: the national death index (DHHS Publication No. PHS 81–1148). Washington (DC): Government Printing Office; 1981.

Norusis MJ: SPSS for Windows: professional statistics user's guide. Release 5.0. Chicago: SPSS; 1996.

Olson CM. Peer review of the biomedical literature. Am J Emerg Med 1990;8:356–358.

Orwell G. Politics and the English language. In: A collection of essays by George Orwell. Garden City (NY): Doubleday; 1954. p. 162–176.

Payne LV. The lively art of writing. River Grove (IL): Follet; 1965. p. 64–68.

Polit-O'Hara DF, Hungler BP. Nursing research: principles and methods. 5th ed. Philadelphia: JB Lippincott; 1995.

Protection of human subjects, 45 C.F.R. Sect 46 (1991). Federal Register 1991;56:28003–28032.

Pruitt BA, Mason AD Jr, Moncrief JA. Hemodynamic changes in the early postburn patient: the influence of fluid administration and of a vasodilator (hydralazine). J Trauma 1971;11:36–46.

Roe A. The making of a scientist. New York: Dodd, Mead; 1953.

Ross PE. Lies, damned lies and medical statistics. Forbes 1995; Aug 14:130–135.

Rothman KJ. Modern epidemiology. Boston: Little, Brown; 1986.

Royall R. Ethics and statistics in randomized clinical trials. Stat Sci 1991;6:52–62.

Sabin WA. The Gregg reference manual. 7th ed. Westerville (OH): Glencoe; 1992.

Sackett DL. Bias in analytic research. J Chronic Dis 1979;32:51–63.

Sackett DL, Haynes RB, Guyatt GH, et al. Clinical epidemiology: a basic science for clinical medicine. 2nd ed. Boston: Little, Brown; 1991.

Salsburg DS. The religion of statistics as practiced in medical journals. Am Stat 1985;39:220–223.

Salzberg CA, Byrne DW, Cayten CG, et al. A new pressure ulcer risk assessment scale for individuals with spinal cord injury. Am J Phys Med Rehabil 1996;75:96–104.

Seeff LB, Buskell-Bales Z, Wright EC, et al. Long-term mortality after transfusion-associated non-A, non-B hepatitis. N Engl J Med 1992;327:1906–1911.

Sheridan DR, Dowdney DL. How to write and publish articles in nursing. New York: Springer; 1986.

Snedecor GW, Cochran WG. Statistical methods. 8th ed. Ames (IA): Iowa State University Press; 1989.

Spilker B. Guide to clinical trials. New York: Raven Press; 1991.

Spilker B, Schoenfelder J. Data collection forms in clinical trials. New York: Raven Press; 1991.

S-Plus for Windows user's manual. Version 3.3. Seattle: MathSoft; 1995. p. 1–53.

Sprinthall RC. Basic statistical analysis. 5th ed. Des Moines: Allyn and Bacon; 1997.

Standards of Reporting Trials Group. A proposal for structured reporting of randomized controlled trials. JAMA 1994;272:1926–1931.

StatXact 3 for Windows user manual. Cambridge (MA): Cytel Software; 1995.

Stedman's medical dictionary. 26th ed. Baltimore: Williams & Wilkins; 1995.

Stein J, Flexner SB, editors. Random House college thesaurus. New York: Random House; 1992.

Strunk W Jr, White EB. The elements of style. 3rd ed. Old Tappan (NJ): Macmillan; 1979.

Testa MA, Simonson DC. Assessment of quality-of-life outcomes. N Engl J Med 1996;334:835–840.

Truog RD. Randomized controlled trials: lessons from ECMO. Clin Res 1992;40:519–527.

US Department of Health and Human Services. Federal policy for the protection of human subjects: notices and rules. Federal Register 1991;46:28001–28032.

US Department of Health and Human Services, Public Health Service: Healthy People 2000 (DHHS Publication No. PHS 91–50212). Washington (DC): Government Printing Office; 1991.

Virchow R. Quoted by Garrison FH in Bulletin of the New York Academy of Medicine 1928;4:94. In: Strauss MB, editor. Familiar medical quotations. Boston: Little, Brown; 1968.

Ware JH, Mosteller F, Ingelfinger JA. P values. In: Bailar JC III, Mosteller F, editors. Medical uses of statistics. 2nd ed. Boston: Massachusetts Medical Society; 1992.

Wilcoxon F. Individual comparisons by ranking methods. Biomed Bull 1945; 1:80–83.

Williams JM. Style: toward clarity and grace. Chicago: University of Chicago Press; 1995.

World Medical Association. Declaration of Helsinki: recommendations guiding physicians in biomedical research involving human subjects. JAMA 1997;227:925–926.

Yancey JM. Ten rules for reading clinical research reports [editorial]. Am J Surg 1990;159:533–539.

Zeger SL, Liang KY. Longitudinal data analysis for discrete and continuous outcomes. Biometrics 1986;42:121–130.

Index

Note: Page numbers in *italic* indicate illustrations; page numbers followed by t indicate tables.

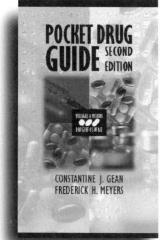
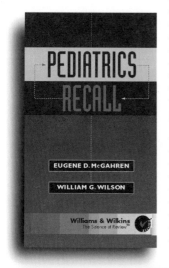
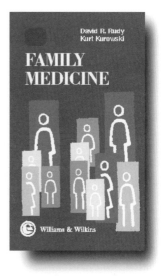